Population-Based Nutrition Epidemiology

Population-Based Nutrition Epidemiology

Editor

Demosthenes Panagiotakos

MDPI • Basel • Beijing • Wuhan • Barcelona • Belgrade • Manchester • Tokyo • Cluj • Tianjin

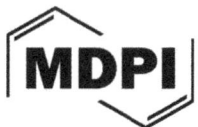

Editor
Demosthenes Panagiotakos
Harokopio University Athens
Greece

Editorial Office
MDPI
St. Alban-Anlage 66
4052 Basel, Switzerland

This is a reprint of articles from the Special Issue published online in the open access journal *Nutrients* (ISSN 2072-6643) (available at: https://www.mdpi.com/journal/nutrients/special_issues/Population_Based_Nutrition_Epidemiology).

For citation purposes, cite each article independently as indicated on the article page online and as indicated below:

LastName, A.A.; LastName, B.B.; LastName, C.C. Article Title. *Journal Name* **Year**, *Volume Number*, Page Range.

ISBN 978-3-0365-0018-8 (Hbk)
ISBN 978-3-0365-0019-5 (PDF)

© 2020 by the authors. Articles in this book are Open Access and distributed under the Creative Commons Attribution (CC BY) license, which allows users to download, copy and build upon published articles, as long as the author and publisher are properly credited, which ensures maximum dissemination and a wider impact of our publications.

The book as a whole is distributed by MDPI under the terms and conditions of the Creative Commons license CC BY-NC-ND.

Contents

About the Editor vii

Demosthenes B. Panagiotakos, Matina Kouvari and Kyriakos Souliotis
Towards a Better Primary Healthcare in Europe: Shifts in Public Health Nutrition Policies
Reprinted from: *Nutrients* 2020, 12, 3308, doi:10.3390/nu12113308 1

Hazzaa M. Al-Hazzaa, Amani A. Al-Rasheedi, Rayan A. Alsulaimani and Laura Jabri
Anthropometric, Familial- and Lifestyle-Related Characteristics of School Children Skipping Breakfast in Jeddah, Saudi Arabia
Reprinted from: *Nutrients* 2020, 12, 3668, doi:10.3390/nu12123668 5

Jasmina B. Timic, Jelena Kotur-Stevuljevic, Heiner Boeing, Dušanka Krajnovic, Brizita Djordjevic and Sladjana Sobajic
A Cross-Sectional Survey of Salty Snack Consumption among Serbian Urban-Living Students and Their Contribution to Salt Intake
Reprinted from: *Nutrients* 2020, 12, 3290, doi:10.3390/nu12113290 25

Yoshiaki Nomura, Yoshimasa Ishii, Shunsuke Suzuki, Kenji Morita, Akira Suzuki, Senichi Suzuki, Joji Tanabe, Yasuo Ishiwata, Koji Yamakawa, Yota Chiba, Meu Ishikawa, Kaoru Sogabe, Erika Kakuta, Ayako Okada, Ryoko Otsuka and Nobuhiro Hanada
Nutritional Status and Oral Frailty: A Community Based Study
Reprinted from: *Nutrients* 2020, 12, 2886, doi:10.3390/nu12092886 39

Matthew R. Jeans, Fiona M. Asigbee, Matthew J. Landry, Sarvenaz Vandyousefi, Reem Ghaddar, Heather J. Leidy and Jaimie N. Davis
Breakfast Consumption in Low-Income Hispanic Elementary School-Aged Children: Associations with Anthropometric, Metabolic, and Dietary Parameters
Reprinted from: *Nutrients* 2020, 12, 2038, doi:10.3390/nu12072038 53

Marzena Jezewska-Zychowicz, Jerzy Gebski and Milena Kobylińska
Food Involvement, Eating Restrictions and Dietary Patterns in Polish Adults: Expected Effects of Their Relationships (LifeStyle Study)
Reprinted from: *Nutrients* 2020, 12, 1200, doi:10.3390/nu12041200 71

Roberta Zupo, Rodolfo Sardone, Rossella Donghia, Fabio Castellana, Luisa Lampignano, Ilaria Bortone, Giovanni Misciagna, Giovanni De Pergola, Francesco Panza, Madia Lozupone, Andrea Passantino, Nicola Veronese, Vito Guerra, Heiner Boeing and Gianluigi Giannelli
Traditional Dietary Patterns and Risk of Mortality in a Longitudinal Cohort of the Salus in Apulia Study
Reprinted from: *Nutrients* 2020, 12, 1070, doi:10.3390/nu12041070 85

Fotios Barkas, Tzortzis Nomikos, Evangelos Liberopoulos and Demosthenes Panagiotakos
Diet and Cardiovascular Disease Risk Among Individuals with Familial Hypercholesterolemia: Systematic Review and Meta-Analysis
Reprinted from: *Nutrients* 2020, 12, 2436, doi:10.3390/nu12082436 101

About the Editor

Demosthenes Panagiotakos (male, born 1967) is a Professor in Biostatistics, Research Methods and Epidemiology at Harokopio University in Athens, Greece. He is also a member of the Scientific Committee of Health, Environment and Emerging Risks/DG Health and Food Safety, of the European Commission (2016–2021). From 2016–2019, he was Vice Rector of Financial Affairs, Research and Development at the University; previously he served as the Dean of the School of Health Sciences & Education (2013–2016). Prof Panagiotakos is also a visiting Distinguished Professor at the School of Arts and Sciences, Rutgers, the State University of New Jersey, USA, and an adjunct professor at the Faculty of Health, University of Canberra, ACT, Australia. As the Principal Investigator, he has supervised 17 large-scale, epidemiological studies and research projects. His research interests include chronic disease epidemiology, medical research methodology, personalized medicine, and risk modeling. He has published 3 books, over 800 scientific papers in peer-reviewed international journals, as well as 50 papers in national journals and conference proceedings and has more than 28,500 citations of his work (h-index of 73). He has received several national and international awards and scholarships. He has served as a research evaluator for National and International Organizations (including the European Commission, JCR, etc.), a reviewer in international journals, and an external evaluator for several faculty positions. He is an Executive Board member in 3 Scientific Societies and former President of the Hellenic Atherosclerosis Society. He serves as an Editor-in-Chief, Associate Editor, or Editorial Board member for 17 international journals. He has been invited to give more than 250 lectures in 17 countries around the world in the field of cardiovascular disease epidemiology and its risk determinants. He has actively participated in campaigns against tobacco use and substances, and exposure to environmental tobacco smoking, as well as promoted healthy dietary patterns and the Mediterranean diet. He is a Board Member of the National Nutrition Policy Committee of the Ministry of Health and has served as a Board Member of the Scientific Council of the Hellenic Food Authority and the National Council of Public Health.

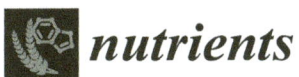

Editorial

Towards a Better Primary Healthcare in Europe: Shifts in Public Health Nutrition Policies

Demosthenes B. Panagiotakos [1,2,*], Matina Kouvari [1] and Kyriakos Souliotis [3]

1. Department of Nutrition and Dietetics, School of Health Science and Education, Harokopio University, 17671 Athens, Greece; matinakouvari4@gmail.com
2. Faculty of Health, University of Canberra, Bruce ACT 2617, Australia
3. Faculty of Social and Political Sciences, University of Peloponnese, 20100 Korinthos, Greece; ksouliotis@uop.gr
* Correspondence: d.b.panagiotakos@usa.net

Received: 15 October 2020; Accepted: 27 October 2020; Published: 29 October 2020

Keywords: health policies; nutrition policies; Europe; primary care

---

The interrelated challenges of suboptimal dietary habits and abnormal weight status have never been as high on the global and European public health agenda as nowadays [1]. Non-communicable diseases (NCDs), including cardiovascular diseases (CVD), cancer, diabetes and respiratory disease, kill 41 million people each year, equivalent to 71% of all deaths and >80% of premature deaths globally [2]. Obesity prevalence is either rapidly increasing or stabilizing at very high levels in almost all European countries [3]. On the other side, the latest results from the ongoing Global Burden of Disease Study revealed that one in five deaths globally can be attributed to an unhealthy diet, with this proportion soaring when abnormal weight status and other measures of maternal and child malnutrition are included [4]. Similarly, it is estimated that among all behaviors, nutrition makes the largest contribution to CVD mortality and morbidity at the population level across Europe [5].

Countries in the World Health Organization (WHO) European Region are rather diverse in terms of income and development levels, as well as food culture and traditions. However, their dietary habits are commonly suboptimal, characterized by energy imbalance and excessive intake of saturated fats, trans fatty acids, added sugars and salt—largely due to increased consumption of highly processed, energy-dense manufactured foods and sugar-sweetened beverages—as well as inadequate consumption of vegetables, fruits and whole grains [6]. Regions of low socioeconomic status are the most severely affected, with major economic and welfare costs for the whole society [7]. Such observations spur the need for ambitious action by European governments.

Comprehensive policies to promote healthy diets and prevent obesity in the European Region have been advocated by the WHO Regional Office for Europe since the adaptation of the first action plan in 2000 [8] (Figure 1). This action plan explicitly called on member states to introduce strategies on food and nutrition so as to reach the European Health21 target regarding healthier living, i.e., "By the year 2015, people across society should have adopted healthier patterns of living" [8]. This first action plan principally focused on the prevention of foodborne diseases as well as nutrition-related socioeconomic inequalities and food insecurity [8]. Since then, one third of the member states in the WHO European Region developed policies on food and nutrition and almost all had government-approved documents dealing with nutrition and food safety [9]. In 2008, a renewed nutrition action plan was launched [10]. This time, the action plan addressed the main public health challenges in the areas of nutrition, food safety and food security, dealing with diet-related NCDs (principally obesity), micronutrient deficiencies and foodborne diseases. A couple of years later, a number of "best buys" including recommended actions on salt and trans-fat consumption or limiting children's exposure to advertising for foods high in saturated fats, sugars and salt were recognized [11].

In 2011, the Regional Committee adopted resolution EUR/RC61/R3 which endorsed the Action Plan for implementation of the European Strategy for the Prevention and Control of Non-communicable Diseases (NCD) 2012–2016 [12]. Three out of five priority interventions were related with "promotion of healthy consumption via fiscal and marketing policies", "elimination of trans fats in food (and their replacement with polyunsaturated fats)" and "salt reduction". In 2013, ministers of countries of the European Region adopted the "Vienna Declaration on Nutrition and Noncommunicable Diseases in the Context of Health 2020". This declaration acknowledged that strategies to improve dietary health require government-led action in a broad range of areas and should be informed by increasing evidence of the efficacy of a comprehensive response incorporating a core set of policies. It also recognized that successful adoption and implementation of these policies requires continuing emphasis on health-in-all-policies and whole-of-government approaches for the creation of healthy and sustainable food systems, in line with the European Health 2020 strategy [13]. Following this, the global action plan for the prevention and control of NCDs was launched, setting a 25% relative reduction in overall mortality of cardiovascular disease, diabetes, cancer and respiratory diseases as well as describing specific nutrition-related targets [14]. To meet this challenge, the European Food and Nutrition Action Plan 2015–2020 was endorsed by member states. This action plan included state-of-the-art knowledge on the factors that influence dietary behavior throughout the life-course and policies and interventions for a wide range of settings and domains [15].

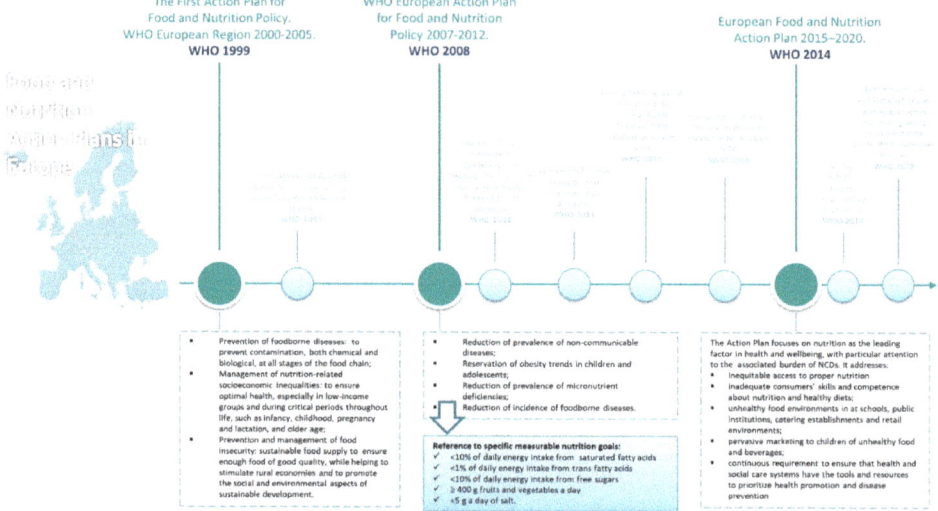

Figure 1. Public health and nutrition policies in Europe. Abbreviations: NCD (non-communicable diseases); WHO (World Health Organization). Source of information included in figure: [8–15].

Within the most recent action plan, member states had to develop common tools, share experiences, improve the availability of data and enhance capacity for monitoring and surveillance so as to halt increases in obesity and diabetes, halt the increase in the prevalence of overweight status among children under five years old, reduce the mean population intake of salt and sodium by 30%, increase the rate of exclusive breastfeeding in the first six months of life to at least 50% and reduce the proportion of stunted children under five years by 40% as well as the prevalence of anemia among non-pregnant women of reproductive age by 50%. All of these have been set as the global nutrition targets for 2025 [16]. Policy options that governments might consider included the creation of healthy food environments from school to food markets. In particular, labelling trans fatty acids content and food and beverage reformulation—to tackle nutrient deficiencies—as well as setting specific regulations regarding the marketing of food products, especially toward children, have been developed. Additionally, the promotion of healthy dietary habits during pregnancy as well as early in life was highlighted. Moreover, this action plan underlined the role of health professionals in offering nutrition counselling, particularly in the primary health care context and the need for public to be provided with nutritional skills and capacity. Finally, surveillance, monitoring and evaluation of the applied policies, including monitoring the growth of children under five years old or assessment of individuals' dietary habits through representative national surveys, were indispensable parts of this action plan [15].

According to the latest report of the European Commission, more than 750,000 deaths per year are attributed to behavioral factors, with nutrition and increased weight status being on the short list [17]. The role of food environments in positively or negatively affecting people's food choices, dietary behavior and, subsequently, health outcomes has been well described in the literature. Nowadays, a suite of policies are recognized as essential for creating a healthy food environment on a national and European basis. The importance of nutrition throughout life-course has been well understood and appreciated to prevent obesity and NCDs. Towards this need, tailor-made policies are demanded to effectively target each different life stage. On the other side, the health system demonstrates a major role in promoting healthy dietary behaviors. In this context, practice and training for health professionals might have to be transformed, including investment in more diversified human resources at primary care level.

All of these are put under the umbrella of primary care strategies. Considering that in the meanwhile, only 3% of total health expenditures in EU Member States is devoted to primary care, many things remain to be done. Besides the fact that significant progress has been made in various areas of public health nutrition, the European Region is not fully on-track to achieve the global NCD targets. Therefore, more ambitious and comprehensive nutrition policies should be prioritized at a faster pace, accompanied by a more robust monitoring system to discriminate progress and to guide timely and effective policies.

Author Contributions: D.B.P. and M.K. performed the review of nutrition policies and summarized the main findings. M.K. wrote the manuscript. D.B.P. and K.S. critically reviewed the manuscript. All authors have read and agreed to the published version of the manuscript.

Funding: This research received no external funding.

Conflicts of Interest: The authors declare no conflict of interest.

References

1. World Health Organization. *Regional Office for Europe Better Food and Nutrition in Europe: A Progress Report Monitoring Policy Implementation in the WHO European Region*; WHO Regional Office for Europe: Copenhagen, Denmark, 2018.
2. World Health Organization. *Global Status Report on Non-Communicable Diseases 2014*; World Health Organization: Geneva, Switzerland, 2014.
3. Abarca-Gómez, L.; Abdeen, Z.A.; Hamid, Z.A.; Abu-Rmeileh, N.M.; Acosta-Cazares, B.; Acuin, C.; Adams, R.J.; Aekplakorn, W.; Afsana, K.; Aguilar-Salinas, C.A.; et al. Worldwide trends in body-mass index, underweight, overweight, and obesity from 1975 to 2016: A pooled analysis of 2416 population-based measurement studies in 128·9 million children, adolescents, and adults. *The Lancet* **2017**, *390*, 2627–2642. [CrossRef]
4. Gakidou, E.; Afshin, A.; Abajobir, A.A.; Abate, K.H.; Abbafati, C.; Abbas, K.M.; Abd-Allah, F.; Abdulle, A.M.; Abera, S.F.; Aboyans, V.; et al. Global, regional, and national comparative risk assessment of 84 behavioural, environmental and occupational, and metabolic risks or clusters of risks, 1990–2016: A systematic analysis for the global burden of disease study 2016. *Lancet* **2017**, *390*, 1345–1422. [CrossRef]
5. Wilkins, E.; Wilson, L.; Wickramasinghe, K.; Bhatnagar, P.; Leal, J.; Luengo-Fernandez, R.; Burns, R.; Rayner, M. *Townsend N European Cardiovascular Disease Statistics 2017*; European Heart Network: Brussels, Belgium, 2017.
6. Breda, J.; Castro, L.S.N.; Whiting, S.; Williams, J.; Jewell, J.; Engesveen, K.; Wickramasinghe, K. Towards better nutrition in Europe: Evaluating progress and defining future directions. *Food Policy* **2020**, 101887. [CrossRef]

7. Turrell, G.; Vandevijvere, S. Socio-economic inequalities in diet and body weight: Evidence, causes and intervention options. *Public Health Nutr.* **2015**, *18*, 759–763. [CrossRef] [PubMed]
8. World Health Organization. *The First Action Plan for Food and Nutrition Policy. WHO European Region 2000–2005*; Nutrition and Food Security Programme Division of Technical Support and Strategic Development; WHO: Geneva, Switzerland, 1999.
9. World Health Organization. *Regional Office for Europe Comparative Analysis of Food and Nutrition Policies in WHO European Member States*; Nutrition and Food Security Programme; WHO: Geneva, Switzerland, 2003.
10. World Health Organization. *WHO European Action Plan for Food and Nutrition Policy 2007–2012*; WHO: Geneva, Switzerland, 2008.
11. World Health Organization. *Moscow Declaration: The First Global Ministerial Conference on Healthy Lifestyles and Noncommunicable Disease Control*; WHO: Moscow, Russia, 2011.
12. World Health Organization. *Global Status Report on Noncommunicable Disease*; WHO: Geneva, Switzerland, 2011.
13. World Health Organization. Regional office for europe vienna declaration on nutrition and noncommunicable diseases in the context of health 2020. In Proceedings of the WHO Ministerial Conference on Nutrition and Noncommunicable Diseases in the Context of Health 2020, Vienna, Austria, 4–5 July 2013.
14. World Health Organization. *Global Action Plan for the Prevention and Control of NCDs 2013–2020*; WHO: Geneva, Switzerland, 2013.
15. World Health Organization. *Regional Office for Europe European Food and Nutrition Action Plan 2015–2020*; World Health Organization, Regional Office for Europe: Geneva, Switzerland, 2015.
16. World Health Organization. *Global Nutrition Targets 2025: Policy Brief Series*; WHO: Geneva, Switzerland, 2014.
17. *European Commission State of Health in the EU: Companion Report 2019*; European Commission: Luxembourg, 2019.

Publisher's Note: MDPI stays neutral with regard to jurisdictional claims in published maps and institutional affiliations.

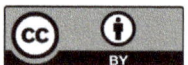

© 2020 by the authors. Licensee MDPI, Basel, Switzerland. This article is an open access article distributed under the terms and conditions of the Creative Commons Attribution (CC BY) license (http://creativecommons.org/licenses/by/4.0/).

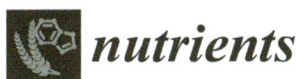

Article

Anthropometric, Familial- and Lifestyle-Related Characteristics of School Children Skipping Breakfast in Jeddah, Saudi Arabia

Hazzaa M. Al-Hazzaa [1,*], Amani A. Al-Rasheedi [2], Rayan A. Alsulaimani [3] and Laura Jabri [4]

1. Lifestyle and Health Research Center, Health Sciences Research Center, Princess Nourah bint Abdulrahman University, Riyadh 11671, Saudi Arabia
2. Food and Nutrition Department, Faculty of Human Sciences and Design, King Abdul Aziz University, Jeddah 42751, Saudi Arabia; aalrasheedi@kau.edu.sa
3. Department of Pharmacology, Faculty of Medicine, King Abdul Aziz University, Jeddah 42751, Saudi Arabia; raalsulaimani@kau.edu.sa
4. American International School of Jeddah, Jeddah 21352, Saudi Arabia; laurajabri@gmail.com
* Correspondence: halhazzaa@hotmail.com

Received: 18 October 2020; Accepted: 26 November 2020; Published: 29 November 2020

Abstract: Breakfast is a vital meal that provides children with important nutrients and energy. This study examined the anthropometric, familial- and lifestyle-related characteristics of school children skipping breakfast. A total of 1149 children (boys: 45.5%), 6 to 12 years old (mean and SD: 9.3 ± 1.7 years), were randomly selected from elementary schools in Jeddah. Weight and height were measured. Breakfast eating frequency, socio-demographics, and lifestyle behaviors were assessed using a specifically designed self-report questionnaire reported by the parents. Nearly 80% of the children skipped daily breakfast at home with no significant age or gender differences. The most common reasons for skipping breakfast at home included not feeling hungry and waking up late for school. Fried egg sandwiches and breakfast cereals were most frequently consumed for breakfast. Strong parental support for breakfast as the main daily meal was significantly associated with daily breakfast intake. Logistic regression analyses, adjusted for age, gender, and socio-demographics, revealed that paternal education (aOR = 1.212, 95% CI = 1.020–1.440, $p = 0.029$), maternal education (aOR = 1.212, 95% CI = 1.003–1.464, $p=0.046$), insufficient sleep (aOR = 0.735, 95% CI = 0.567–0.951, $p = 0.019$), and BMI <25 kg/m^2 (aOR = 1.333, 95% CI = 1.015–1.752, $p = 0.039$) were significantly associated with breakfast intake. The findings have implications for children's health and school performance. Concerted effort is required to promote breakfast consumption among Saudi children.

Keywords: breakfast intake; children; lifestyle behaviors; obesity; sociodemographic factors

1. Introduction

Childhood obesity continues to be a global public health concern, along with its associated rise in cardiometabolic complications [1]. Meta-analysis research and a systematic review revealed that childhood overweight or obesity tracks well into adulthood, with 55% of obese children becoming obese adolescents and 80% of obese adolescents remaining obese in adulthood [2]. Worldwide, the prevalence of overweight and obesity among school-aged children and adolescents has risen enormously over the past decades [3]. In Saudi Arabia, a recent study conducted in Riyadh indicated that the prevalence of overweight plus obesity among children 6–8 years old and 9–11 years old were 24.6% and 30.9%, respectively [4]. Well-recognized major modifiable determinants of childhood obesity include diet and physical activity [5]. Although genetic factors may influence predisposition to obesity, a healthy—as opposed to unhealthy—lifestyle was reported to substantially lower the risk of obesity by 85% among children at high polygenic risk [6].

Regular breakfast intake in children has been shown to be associated with healthy body weight [7]. Numerous studies have indicated that skipping breakfast predisposes children and adolescents to obesity [8–11]. In one North American study, adolescents who consumed breakfast more often had a lower body mass index (BMI) than those who skipped breakfast [8]. In prospective analyses, frequency of breakfast intake among children from the USA was inversely associated with BMI in a dose-response manner [12]. Further, in longitudinal research from Japan, it was shown that skipping breakfast in early childhood increased overweight/obesity in later childhood [13]. In another longitudinal study involving Croatian adolescents, participants who consumed breakfast had significantly lower body fat percentages compared to those who skipped breakfast [14]. Local studies regarding breakfast and overweight or obesity status among Saudi children showed conflicting results [15,16]. While one study found that the majority of the underweight (94%) and obese children (89%) reported skipping breakfast [15], another recent study found no association between obesity level and breakfast consumption [16]. Different methods of sampling and calculating obesity status may have contributed for the differences in their results. Nevertheless, it is well recognized that the association between breakfast intake and obesity is confounded by many factors, including socioeconomic factors, home environment, circadian rhythms, and a variety of lifestyle behaviors such as eating fast food, physical activity and sedentary lifestyle [17].

Breakfast is a vital meal that provides children with important nutrients and energy. Consuming breakfast can improve cognitive learning and academic performance among children and adolescents [18–20]. In addition, children who skip breakfast have less healthful diets than children who regularly consume breakfast. Skipping breakfast was shown to disturb the adequacy of nutrient intake in a recent multicenter European study involving a large number of adolescents from ten cities [21]. It was also found that skipping breakfast leads to poorer diet quality among children and adolescents [22]. In addition, among Lebanese adolescents, skipping breakfast was associated with lower adherence to the Mediterranean diet [23].

Although regular breakfast consumption can have a multitude of positive health benefits, Saudi children were found to be more likely to skip breakfast than any other meal. A recent study on daily breakfast intake among Saudi children in Riyadh indicated that skipping an at-home breakfast has reached nearly 80% [16]. Skipping breakfast was found to be associated with insufficient sleep duration among Saudi children [24]. Furthermore, unhealthy lifestyle behaviors were shown to be negatively associated with daily breakfast behaviors in the Health Behaviour in School-aged Children study [25]. The high prevalence rate for skipping breakfast at home reported by children and adolescents in Saudi Arabia is very alarming and deserves further investigation [15,16,26–28]. Understanding the important familial, sociodemographic, and lifestyle determinants of breakfast consumption can also help in recognizing children at risk of skipping breakfast and may enhance our ability to plan and implement effective programs for preventing unhealthy breakfast intake behaviors in children. Therefore, in the present study, we report on the anthropometric, familial- and lifestyle-related characteristics among primary school children living in Jeddah, Saudi Arabia, relative to breakfast intake frequency and describe breakfast intake preferences by Saudi children relative to gender.

2. Materials and Methods

2.1. Study Design and Sample Selection

This is a cross-sectional study that was conducted in Jeddah during the 2019 school year. Jeddah, the second most populated city in Saudi Arabia, has a multiethnic population with over three million inhabitants. All Saudi children enrolled in boys' and girls' elementary schools from grades 1–6 during the study period were eligible for inclusion in the study. The exception was if the child had a medical condition related to eating disorders. In Saudi Arabia, schooling in grades 1–12 is mandatory and offered for free in public schools. The sample size was calculated with the assumption that the population proportion would yield the maximum possible sample size required (proportion = 0.50), with a confidence level of 95% and a margin of error of 4%. An additional 20% of participants were added to account for non-responders, or missing data. The total sample size for each gender was calculated to be 480 children, with 960 boys and girls in total.

A representative random sample was selected from schools using a multistage stratified cluster sampling technique. Stratification was based on boys' and girls' schools (boys' and girls' schools are segregated in Saudi Arabia), public and private schools, as well as on major geographical locations (east, west, north, and south). Children were drawn from elementary schools relative to the actual number of students in public and private schools and geographical location in Jeddah. Within each area, one private and two public schools were randomly selected. Then, within each school, a class was randomly selected from each of the six grades. The final number of classes selected from all six grades was 72. All Saudi students in the designated classes were then invited to participate in the study. Figure 1 illustrates the protocol that was used for the students' selection. Normally, there are about 25 Saudi students in each class in public schools and nearly 15 Saudi students in each class in private schools. Ethical approval was obtained from the Institutional Review Board (IRB) at Princess Nourah bint Abdulrahman University, Riyadh (IRB Log Number: 19-0014). The research procedures were conducted in accordance with the principles expressed in the Declaration of Helsinki. Written informed consent was obtained from all participating parents. Approval for conducting this research in schools was secured from the Jeddah directorate of schools, Ministry of Education, and the principals of the selected schools.

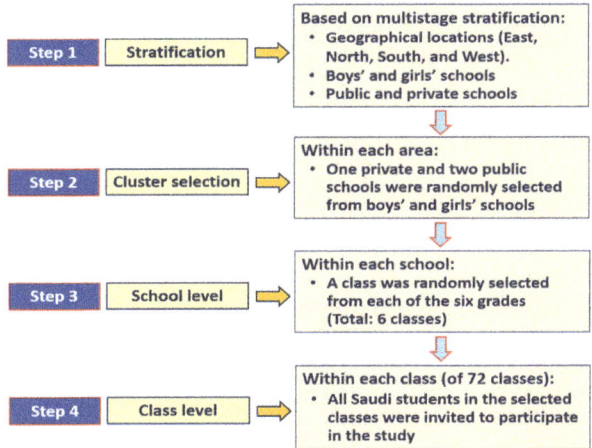

Figure 1. The protocol used for participants' selection.

2.2. Anthropometric Measurement

Body weight was measured to the nearest 100 g using calibrated portable medical scales (Seca 869, Birmingham, UK). All measurements were taken with minimal clothing and without shoes by trained researchers. Height was measured to the nearest 0.1 cm using a measuring rod calibrated to the nearest centimeter while the subject was in a full standing position without shoes. Body mass index (BMI) was computed as the ratio of weight in kilograms divided by the squared height in meters. The extended International Obesity Task Force (IOTF) age- and sex-specific BMI cutoff reference standards were used to classify underweight, normal weight, and overweight or obesity relative to the child's age [29].

2.3. Assessment of Breakfast Eating Habits

Breakfast eating habits and food preferences were assessed using a specifically designed self-report questionnaire that was filled out by the children's parents [16]. With clear instructions, parents were asked to complete the questionnaire forms based on the child's typical (habitual) breakfast habits. In addition, the questionnaire form included information on demographic and socioeconomic status. Additional questions were related to breakfast choices and behaviors as well as how satisfied the parents were with their child's breakfast choices (three Likert scale; satisfied, somewhat satisfied, or not satisfied) and the level of importance of breakfast intake as a meal for their child (very important, somewhat important, or not important). A variety of common breakfast choices were provided in the questionnaire, including cheese, eggs, ready-to-eat cereals, pizza, peanut butter or hummus sandwiches, potatoes, sausage, cookies, and muffins. The questionnaire was previously developed and content validated and reviewed and agreed upon by three experts in the field of nutrition and dietary habits [16]. The actual questionnaire can be found as a supplementary file in a previous publication [16].

2.4. Assessment of Screen Time, Sleep, and Physical Activity

Assessment of screen time, sleep, and physical activity was part of the breakfast intake questionnaire. Questions related to screen time included items intended to determine information from the parents about the typical amount of daily screen time the child spent, including time spent watching TV, playing non-active video games, and using the computer and internet for recreational purposes. Parents were asked to provide the average usual hours spent during weekdays and weekends. For classifying screen time cutoff hours, we used the American Academy of Pediatrics guidelines and the Canadian 24-Hour Movement Guidelines for Children and Youth (ages 5–17 years) which call for a maximum of two hours per day of screen time [30,31].

Nocturnal sleep duration on weekdays (school days) and weekends was assessed using questions embedded within the questionnaire. Parents were asked how many hours their children usually sleep at night on weekdays and weekends. We defined insufficient sleep (short sleepers) as sleeping less than nine hours per night, according to the definition of the National Sleep Foundation for school-age children 6 to 13 years old [32].

Physical activity was assessed using the total daily time spent by the child on all types of physical activities, including sports, during which the child's breathing was considerably increased. The sufficient physical activity level was based on 60 min or more of daily physical activity [33]. Accordingly, physical activity was classified as low or high activity based on a cutoff value of 420 min per week or the recommended daily time for children and adolescents [31,33].

2.5. Statistical Analysis

Data were entered into an SPSS data file, checked, cleaned, and analyzed using the IBM-SPSS software, version 22 (Chicago, IL, USA). Descriptive statistics were obtained for all variables and reported as means and standard deviations or percentages. Differences between boys and girls in selected descriptive measurements were tested using MANCOVA tests while controlling for socioeconomic status. Bonferroni test was used for testing in-between subject differences. Chi-square tests of proportions were used to test differences in sociodemographic factors and dichotomized lifestyle behaviors. Multivariable analyses (MANCOVA) were used to test differences in selected variables (gender and frequency of breakfast intake (below 5 days per week versus 5 or more days per week)) while controlling for age and sociodemographic factors. Since physical activity in minutes per week is not normally distributed, we used log transformation when analyzing physical activity in the MANCOV test. Wilks' Lambda tests as multivariable test was reported as well as tests of between subject's effects (Bonferroni test) for breakfast intake, gender, and the interactions of breakfast intake with gender. Finally, logistic regression analysis of selected lifestyle behaviors was used to test differences in the frequency breakfast intake (high versus low intake) among Saudi children, while adjusted for age, gender, and sociodemographic factors. Adjusted odds ratios (aOR) and confidence intervals (95% CI) were reported. Alpha level was set at 0.05, and p-value less than alpha level was considered significant.

3. Results

Table 1 displays the descriptive characteristics of the participants. The total number of the sample was 1,149 children (523 boys and 626 girls) between the ages of 6 and 13 with a mean age (SD) of 9.2 (1.7) years. No significant ($p = 0.365$) difference in age was observed between boys and girls. There were no significant differences between boys and girls in body weight ($p = 0.246$), height ($p = 0.608$), or BMI value ($p = 0.055$). Breakfast intake averaged 3.76 ± 2.3 days per week, with no significant ($p = 0.778$) differences between boys and girls. In addition, there were no significant differences between boys and girls in breakfast intake on weekdays ($p = 0.809$) or weekends ($p = 0.793$). The findings also showed that the prevalence of children having daily breakfast at home was 20.4%. The most noted reasons for those children not regularly having breakfast at home included the child not feeling hungry (47.6%), the child waking up late and not having time for breakfast at home (in which case, he/she was given a sandwich to eat on the way to school or at school) (36.1%), and the child being given money to buy food from the school canteen (26.7%). Furthermore, BMI classifications showed no significant ($p = 0.093$) difference between boys and girls in the proportions of underweight, normal weight, and overweight or obesity. The prevalence of overweight plus obesity for the entire sample reached 28.7%, with no significant differences relative to gender.

Table 1. Descriptive characteristics of the participants relative to gender.

Variable	All (N = 1149)	Boys (N = 523)	Girls (N = 626)	p-Value *
Age (year)	9.3 ± 1.7	9.3 ± 1.6	9.4 ± 1.7	0.365
Body weight (kg)	32.8 ± 11.3	32.4 ± 11.1	33.2 ± 11.5	0.246
Body height (cm)	133.2 ± 11.4	133.3 ± 10.5	133.0 ± 12.1	0.608
Body mass index (kg/m^2)	18.1 ± 3.9	17.8 ± 4.0	18.3 ± 3.9	0.055
Breakfast intake (days/week)	3.76 ± 2.3	3.75 ± 2.3	3.76 ± 2.2	0.778
BMI category (%)				0.093
Underweight	15.4	17.9	13.3	
Normal weight	55.9	54.7	56.9	
Overweight	19.4	17.5	21.1	
Obesity	9.3	10.0	8.8	
Overweight + obesity	28.7	27.5	29.8	

Data are means ± standard deviations or percentage. * MANCOVA tests while controlling for socioeconomic status (Wilks' Lambda for gender = 0.017). Chi Squares tests for the differences in proportions (BMI category).

The proportions (%) of Saudi children who exceeded certain cutoff values for breakfast intake, overweight/obesity, and selected lifestyle behaviors are presented in Table 2. Nearly 80% of the children did not consume a daily breakfast at home. Almost 70% of the children spent more than two hours of daily screen time, with boys being exceedingly more sedentary than girls. About 66% of the sample did not sleep for the proper duration at night (9 or more hours per night). In addition, the majority (84.8%) of the children were considerably less active than the recommended daily time for physical activity, which amounts to one hour of daily physical activity, with girls having significantly ($p < 0.001$) less physical activity levels than boys. A very small proportion (less than 5%) of the children walked to school.

Table 3 presents the sociodemographic and lifestyle factors of the participants in relation to the breakfast intake category (daily versus non-daily intake). There were no significant differences between children having breakfast for 5 or more days per week compared to those having breakfast for less than 5 days per week in many of the sociodemographic variables, such as gender, school type, parent answering the questionnaire, size of the family living in the house, maternal age, or family income. However, daily breakfast intake appears to associate significantly with lower paternal age, and higher paternal education status. In addition, daily breakfast intake is associated with sleeping sufficiently.

Table 2. The proportions (%) of Saudi children who exceeded certain cut-off values for breakfast intake, overweight/obesity, and selected lifestyle behaviors.

Variable	Criterion *	Proportion (%)			p-Value **
		All (N =1149)	Boys (N = 523)	Girls (N = 626)	
Breakfast intake at home	Non-daily intake	79.6	78.8	80.4	0.509
Overweight or obesity	BMI > cut-offs	28.7	27.5	29.8	0.378
Screen time	>2 h/day	69.5	77.8	62.6	**<0.001**
Nocturnal sleep duration	<9 h	65.8	67.5	64.4	0.267
Physical activity	<420 min/week	84.8	74.8	93.1	**<0.001**
Walking to school	Not walking to school	95.7	95.0	96.3	**0.005**

* Overweight or obesity cut-offs are based on IOTF cut-off values [29], screen time cut-offs are based on reference [30,31], sleep duration cut-offs are based on [32], and physical activity cut-offs are based on [33]; ** Tests for the differences in proportions between boys and girls.

Table 3. Socio-demographic and lifestyle factors of the participants relative to high versus low breakfast intake frequency.

Variable	<5 Days/Week (N = 685)	5 + Days/Week (N = 464)	p-Value *
Breakfast intake (day per week)	2.1 ± 1.1	6.3 ± 0.83	
Gender (%)			0.923
Boys	45.4	45.7	
Girls	54.6	54.3	
School type (%)			0.490
Public	76.4	74.6	
Private	23.6	25.4	
Parent answering the questionnaire (%)			0.099
Father	38.5	33.4	
Mother	58.1	64.2	
Someone else	3.4	2.4	
Number of children in the family (%)			**0.019**
1–2	14.2	18.3	
3–4	49.9	53.0	
5+	35.9	28.7	
Number of family members in the house (%)			0.272
1–3	45.7	50.0	
4–5	50.9	47.6	
6+	3.4	2.4	
Paternal age (%)			**0.019**
<30 years	0.7	0.4	
30-39 years	28.8	32.5	
40–49 years	47.2	51.3	
50–59 years	19.0	13.4	
60+ years	3.4	2.4	
Maternal age (%)			0.057
<30 years	8.2	9.1	
30–39 years	60.3	64.4	
40–49 years	27.2	24.8	
50–59 years	4.4	1.7	
60+ years	0.00	0.00	
Paternal education (%)			**0.001**
Intermediate or less	15.2	9.3	
High school	30.8	25.4	
University degree	46.1	54.3	
Post graduate degree	7.9	11.0	
Maternal education (%)			**<0.001**

Table 3. Cont.

Variable	<5 Days/Week (N = 685)	5 + Days/Week (N = 464)	p-Value *
Intermediate or less	14.0	6.9	
High school	30.2	28.2	
University degree	52.3	59.5	
Post graduate degree	3.5	5.4	
Family income (%) **			0.146
10,000 SR or less	45.8	42.5	
10,001–20,000 SR	37.8	41.2	
20,001–30,000 SR	11.2	13.4	
30,001 + SR	5.1	3.0	
Screen time			0.728
≤2 h/day	30.1	31.0	
>2 h/day	69.9	69.0	
Sleep duration			0.001
<9 h/night	69.5	60.3	
≥9 h/night	30.5	39.7	
Physical activity (%)			0.840
No physical activity	53.1	50.9	
Less than 30 min/day	20.6	21.6	
30 min to less than 60 min/day	11.8	11.2	
60 min/day	8.3	10.6	
More than 60 min/day	3.5	3.4	
Physical activity/inactivity (%)			0.372
Low active	85.5	83.6	
High active	14.5	16.4	
Means of travelling to school (%)			0.291
Walking	4.8	3.4	
Family or private car	86.9	89.9	
School bus	8.3	6.7	
BMI category			0.057
<25 kg/m^2	69.1	74.3	
25 + kg/m^2	30.9	25.7	

* Chi-Square tests for the differences in proportions between daily and non-daily breakfast intake; ** SR = Saudi Riyal = 3.75 U$.

The types of breakfast choices (%) consumed at home by Saudi children relative to gender are shown in Table 4. Varied foods were consumed during breakfast by the Saudi children; however, fried egg sandwiches (48.1%), breakfast cereals (45.9%), and spread cheese sandwiches (41.3%) were the foods most frequently consumed for breakfast, followed by boiled egg sandwiches (27.7%), tuna sandwiches (25.8%), and Nutella sandwiches (25.0%). Healthy breakfast choices, such as falafel sandwiches, thyme pie, labneh pie, and chickpea sandwiches were consumed less frequently (4–7%). Breakfast choices that were consumed significantly more often (for 5 or more days per week compared to less than 5 days per week) included cereals (58.1%), boiled egg sandwiches (32.9%), labneh sandwiches (21.4%), peanut butter sandwiches (12.4%), and solid cheese sandwiches (11.1%).

Table 5 displays breakfast intake preferences by Saudi children relative to gender. Two thirds of the sample preferred to eat breakfast cereals with sugar, whereas nearly 16% preferred cereals with fruit, without any significant difference between boys and girls. Moreover, a higher percentage of boys (60.6%) than girls (46.8%) consumed fresh fruit at breakfast. Apples (31.8%) and bananas (24.6%) were the most consumed fruits for breakfast. Full fat milk (44.6%), water (42.2%), chocolate milk (31.6%), fruit juice (29.4%), and tea with milk (27.2%) were the most common breakfast drinks consumed by the children. Girls showed significantly ($p = 0.003$) higher chocolate milk intake at breakfast than boys. Full fat milk was associated with daily breakfast intake, while chocolate milk was associated with non-breakfast consumption. In addition, there was no association between fruit intake and daily breakfast consumption (not shown in the table).

Table 4. Types of breakfast (%) eaten at home by Saudi children in relation to relative to high versus low breakfast intake frequency (more than one choice was possible).

Variable	Breakfast Intake			p-Value *
	All (N = 1149)	<5 Days/Week (N = 685)	5 + Days/Week (N = 464)	
Fried egg sandwich	48.1	46.1	51.1	0.100
Breakfast cereals	45.9	39.0	56.0	<0.001
Spread cheese sandwich	41.3	39.3	44.4	0.083
Boiled egg sandwich	27.7	25.5	30.8	0.050
Tuna sandwich	25.8	23.9	28.4	0.087
Nutella sandwich	25.0	23.4	27.4	0.123
Croissant	20.3	21.3	18.8	0.289
Labneh sandwich **	16.5	14.2	20.0	0.008
Cheese pie (Fataer Jubin)	14.2	15.2	12.7	0.240
Pancake	13.3	13.9	12.5	0.503
Fava beans (Foul)	12.7	13.0	12.3	0.724
Peanut butter sandwich	8.3	6.7	10.6	0.020
Thyme sandwich	7.8	7.3	8.6	0.413
Cake or cookies	7.6	7.4	7.8	0.844
Pizza	7.6	7.3	8.0	0.671
Mortadella sandwich	7.4	8.5	5.8	0.092
Solid cheese sandwich	7.4	5.5	10.1	0.004
Oreo biscuit/other types of biscuit	7.2	6.7	8.0	0.419
Falafel sandwich	6.9	7.4	6.0	0.354
Jam sandwich	6.6	5.7	8.0	0.127
Thyme pie (Fataer Zatar)	6.4	6.6	6.0	0.715
Labneh pie (Fataer Labneh)	6.4	6.0	6.9	0.534
Hot dog	5.5	6.7	3.7	0.026
Yogurt-with or without fruits	4.6	4.4	5.0	0.647
Chickpeas (Hummus) sandwich	4.2	3.9	4.5	0.627
Other kinds of breakfast ***	12.4	9.9	16.2	0.002

* Chi Squares tests of the proportions for significant difference between frequency of breakfast intake; ** Soft, cream cheese made from strained yogurt, popular in Middle Eastern cuisine; *** Below 4% and include French fries, baked potato, donuts, hamburger, lentils, sweet Arabic pastry, or honey sandwich.

Table 5. Some breakfast intake preferences at home by Saudi children relative to gender (more than one choice was possible).

Variable	All (N = (1149)	Boys (N = (523)	Girls (N = (626)	p-Value *
Preference for cereal with/without added sugar (%)				0.194
With sugar	66.9	65.3	68.1	
Without sugar	33.1	34.7	31.9	
Preference for cereal with or without fruit (%)				0.700
With fruit	15.6	14.6	16.5	
Without fruit	84.4	85.4	83.5	
Percentage of fresh fruit eaten with breakfast (%)	53.1	60.6	46.8	<0.001
Types of fruits consumed most with breakfast (%):				
Apple	31.8	26.8	35.9	0.001
Banana	24.6	26.0	22.9	0.237
Grape	16.6	12.4	20.1	<0.001
Orange	15.9	14.5	17.1	0.237
Strawberries	8.6	3.8	12.6	<0.001
Pear	5.3	6.4	4.0	0.074
Mango	1.8	1.7	1.9	0.805
Kiwi	1.5	1.5	1.4	0.898
Watermelon	1.0	1.0	1.0	0.997
All others (less than 1% each and include dates, pineapple, figs and raisins)	1.1	0.3	2.0	<0.001
Drinks consumed with breakfast (%)	90.5	95.0	86.7	<0.001
Types of Drinks consumed with breakfast (%):				
Full fat milk	44.6	44.0	45.2	0.676

Table 5. Cont.

Variable	All (N = (1149)	Boys (N = (523)	Girls (N = (626)	p-Value *
Water	42.2	39.2	44.7	0.095
Chocolate milk	31.6	27.2	35.3	**0.003**
Fruit juice	29.4	27.3	31.2	0.158
Tea with milk	27.2	28.7	25.9	0.279
Tea	11.6	13.8	9.7	**0.034**
Strawberry milk	9.7	6.7	12.3	**0.001**
Fruit drink	9.4	8.8	9.9	0.521
Low fat milk	8.2	9.4	7.2	0.179
Soft drink (soft beverage)	2.0	3.3	1.0	**0.006**
Butter milk	1.0	1.3	0.8	0.370
Coffee with milk	0.7	1.0	0.5	0.333
Other drinks	1.0	0.0	1.9	0.333

* Chi Squares tests of the proportions for significant difference between males and females.

As shown in Table 6, mothers appear to prepare breakfast nearly 78% of the time, followed by domestic helpers (7.3%). Less than 2% of the children have lactose intolerance. In addition, about 46% of the parents were satisfied with their children's breakfast intake. Parents placed high importance (93.0%) on the breakfast intake of their children, and this significantly impacted the children's daily breakfast intake. Compared to lunch and dinner, 80.6% of parents regarded breakfast as the most important meal of the day for their children, and children with more frequent breakfast intake seemed to have parents with the strongest ($p = 0.024$) opinions on breakfast as the main meal of the day.

Table 6. Factors related to breakfast intake and parent's perception of child's breakfast consumption relative to breakfast intake frequency.

Variable	Frequency of Breakfast Intake			p-Value *
	All (N = 1149)	<5 Days/Week (N = 685)	5 + Days/Week (N = 464)	
Who prepare the breakfast the most for the child? (%)				0.019
Mother	77.9	76.8	79.5	
Domestic helper	7.3	7.0	7.8	
The child himself/herself	4.4	5.8	2.4	
Father	3.6	3.5	3.7	
Nothing is prepared at home	3.0	3.8	1.9	
Sister/brother	2.2	1.5	3.2	
Brought ready from the market	1.6	1.6	1.5	
Does your child have lactose intolerance? (%)				0.266
Yes	1.8	2.2	1.3	
No	98.2	97.8	98.7	
Are you satisfied with the breakfast consumed by your child at home? (%)				0.001
Yes, satisfied	45.7	43.4	49.1	
Somewhat satisfied	46.7	46.7	46.8	
Not satisfied	7.6	9.9	4.1	
As a meal, how important for you is your child's breakfast? (%)				0.069
Very important	93.0	91.5	95.0	
Somewhat important	6.6	7.9	4.7	
Not important	0.4	0.6	0.2	
In your opinion, which is the most important meal of the day for your child? (%)				0.009
Breakfast	80.6	77.7	84.9	
Lunch	17.6	20.1	13.8	
Dinner	1.8	2.2	1.3	

* Chi Squares tests of the proportions for significant difference between daily and non-daily breakfast intake.

Table 7 shows the results of the multivariable analysis of selected anthropometric and lifestyle variables stratified by gender and frequency of breakfast intake (5 or more days per week compared to less than 5 days per week), while controlling for age and socio-demographic factors. There were significant differences in body weight, BMI, and sleep duration between children having more frequent breakfast intake versus less frequent breakfast intake, while there were significant differences relative to gender in screen time, sleep duration, and physical activity levels. In addition, the results of the logistic regression analyses of selected lifestyle behaviors relative to the frequency of breakfast intake, while adjusted for age, gender, and socio-demographic factors, are presented in Table 8. Father's education status (aOR = 1.212, 95% CI = 1.020–1.440, p = 0.029), mother's education (aOR = 1.212, 95% CI = 1.003–1.464, p = 0.046), insufficient sleep duration (aOR = 0.735, 95% CI = 0.567–0.951, p = 0.019), BMI status less than 25 kg/m^2 (aOR = 1.333, 95% CI = 1.015–1.752, p = 0.039) were significantly associated higher frequency of breakfast intake. In another logistic regression model (not shown in a table), we included the type of breakfast choices as independent variables and the results showed that the following breakfast choices were associated with breakfast intake: breakfast cereal (aOR = 1.787, 95% CI = 1.384–2.308, p < 0.001), solid cheese sandwich (aOR = 1.684, 95% CI = 1.050–2.700, p = 0.031), and hot dog (aOR = 0.473, 95% CI = 0.259–0.866, p = 0.015).

Table 7. Multivariate analysis for selected anthropometric and lifestyle variables while controlling for age and socio-demographic factors stratified by gender and breakfast intake frequency. Data are means and standard deviations.

| Variable | Gender | Breakfast Intakes | | p-Value * |
		<5 Days/Week (N = 685)	5 + Days/Week (N = 464)	
Body weight (kg)	Boys	33.5 ± 11.8	30.9 ± 9.6	Breakfast intake: **0.004**
				Gender: 0.287
	Girls	33.8 ± 11.7	32.4 ± 11.3	Breakfast intake by gender interaction: 0.127
	All	33.7 ± 11.8	31.7 ± 10.5	
BMI (kg/m^2)	Boys	18.2 ± 4.2	17.3 ± 3.6	Breakfast intake: **0.009**
	Girls	18.4 ± 3.9	18.0 ± 3.9	Gender: 0.054
	All	18.3 ± 4.0	17.7 ± 3.8	Breakfast intake by gender interaction: 0.213
Screen time (h/night)	Boys	3.55 ± 1.8	3.04 ± 1.5	Breakfast intake: 0.081
				Gender: **<0.001**
	Girls	2.78 ± 1.5	2.81 ± 1.8	Breakfast intake by gender interaction: **0.005**
	All	3.13 ± 1.7	2.91 ± 1.7	Breakfast intake: **<0.001**
Sleep duration (h/night)	Boys	8.18 ± 1.2	8.51 ± 1.1	Gender: **0.025**
	Girls	8.30 ± 1.3	8.63 ± 1.0	Breakfast intake by gender interaction: 0.886
	All	8.25 ± 1.2	8.57 ± 1.1	
Physical activity (min/week)	Boys	196.0 ± 232.5	213.3 ± 225.5	Breakfast intake: 0.526
	Girls	95.2 ± 158.4	92.4 ± 157.8	Gender: **<0.001**
	All	141.2 ± 202.0	148.2 ± 201.1	Breakfast intake by gender interaction: 0.268

* Wilks' Lambda p values: age <0.001; father age = 0.030; mother age = 0.048; father education = 0.002; mother education = 0.135; family income = 0.100; breakfast intake <0.001; gender <0.001 and breakfast intake by gender interaction = 0.056.

Table 8. Results of logistic regression analysis of selected lifestyle behaviors and overweight/obesity status relative to high versus low breakfast intake frequency among Saudi children, while adjusted for age, gender, and socio-demographic factors ($N = 1138$).

Variable	Breakfast Intake (<5 Days/Week Versus 5 + Days/Week) *			
	aOR	(95% CI)	SEE	p-Value
Age	1.008	0.934–1.088	0.039	0.837
Gender (girls = ref)	1.00			
Boys	1.026	0.79401.326	0.131	0.843
No. of family member in the house (high = ref)	1.00			
Low number	1.053	0.797–1.392	0.142	0.715
Paternal age (older age = ref)	1.00			
Younger age	0.937	0.774–1.135	0.098	0.507
Maternal age (older age = ref)	1.00			
younger age	0.953	0.755–1.202	0.119	0.684
Paternal education (high = ref)	1.00			
Low education	1.212	1.020–1.440	0.088	**0.029**
Maternal education (high = ref)	1.00			
Low education	1.212	1.003–1.464	0.096	**0.046**
Family income (> low = ref)	1.00			
High income	0.964	0.808–1.151	0.090	0.688
No. of children in the family (high = ref)	1.00			
Low number of children	0.848	0.673–1.069	0.118	0.163
Screen time (high = ref)	1.00			
Low screen time	1.026	0.784–1.344	0.138	0.849
Sleep duration (sufficient = ref)	1.00			
Insufficient sleep	0.735	0.567–0.951	0.132	**0.019**
Physical activity (active = ref)	1.00			
Inactive	0.899	0.636–1.271	0.177	0.548
Overweight or obesity (BMI ≥ 25 kg/m^2 = ref)	1.00			
BMI < 25 kg/m^2	1.333	1.015–1.752	0.139	**0.039**

* Less than 5 days/week of breakfast intake was used as a reference category. aOR = adjusted odds ratio; CI = confidence interval; ref = reference category; SEE = standard error.

4. Discussion

The present study examined the anthropometric, familial- and lifestyle-related characteristics of Saudi primary school children relative to breakfast intake frequency in Jeddah, Saudi Arabia. The main findings indicated that nearly 80% of the children in this study skipped daily breakfast at home with no significant gender differences. The most common reasons for not having breakfast at home include not being hungry and waking up late for school. In addition, daily breakfast intake appears to associate significantly with the parental and maternal education status, getting sufficient nocturnal sleep, and having normal weight. Fried egg sandwiches, breakfast cereals, and spread cheese sandwiches were the foods most frequently consumed for breakfast. Further, strong parental support of breakfast as the main meal of the day was significantly associated with the child's daily breakfast intake. Finally, logistic regression analysis adjusted for age, gender, and sociodemographic factors indicated that the parental and maternal education status, sufficient sleep duration, and having a BMI value less than 25 kg/m^2 were significantly associated with more frequent child's breakfast intake.

The prevalence of children having daily breakfast at home in the present study was 20.4%, without significant differences relative to age or gender. These findings corroborated recent findings on breakfast consumption (20.7%) reported for primary school children in another major city of the country, Riyadh [16]. However, other earlier studies showed varied breakfast skipping rates. For instance, a small ($n = 120$) study conducted in Riyadh reported that 40.8% of Saudi schoolgirls aged 9 to 13.9 years consumed a daily breakfast and that skipping breakfast increased with advancing age and among children with obesity compared to those without obesity [28]. Among primary students in Abha, in the southern area of Saudi Arabia, breakfast intake was reported as a regular meal for

72% of the children [34]. Moreover, the prevalence of skipping breakfast among male school children from the northern region of Saudi Arabia was reported to be 33.5% [35]. However, in a more recent cross-sectional study ($n = 384$) involving female primary school students from Riyadh, only 2% of the school girls consumed breakfast 5 to 7 days a week [15]. In the current study, more than 40% of our sample consumed breakfast for 5 or more days per week. The differences in the prevalence of breakfast consumption or breakfast skipping rate among Saudi children reported in the above cited studies may generally reflect different questionnaire designs, a small sample size in some studies, or unintended recruitment bias of selected children in other studies.

Elsewhere, the findings from the Health Behaviour in School-aged Children study (HBSC), which included participants from 41 countries, indicated that daily breakfast intake varied from 33% for Greek girls to 75% for Portuguese boys and that low breakfast intake was found in girls and children living in single parent households in many of the participating countries [25]. Furthermore, a lower rate of skipping breakfast was reported among Australian children between the ages of 2 and 17, and skipping breakfast was associated with being female, older, underweight or overweight/obese, and having lower physical activity, inadequate sleep, lower household income, socio-economical disadvantages, and living in a single-parent home [36]. In a study conducted in eight European countries, daily breakfast consumption reported by children varied from 56% in Slovenia to 92% in Spain on weekdays and from 79% in Greece to 93% in Norway on weekends [37]. Among a large group of Greek school children aged 7 to 18 years, 22.4% of boys and 23.1% of girls skipped breakfast [38]. In Bangkok, Thailand, 79% of elementary school children consumed breakfast every day [39].

The findings from the current study showed that logistic regression analysis, while adjusted for age, gender, and sociodemographic factors, indicated that children with BMI value lower than 25 kg/m^2 was significantly associated with more frequent breakfast intake. Local studies regarding breakfast and overweight or obesity status showed conflicting results. While one study found that the majority of the underweight (94%) and obese children (89%) reported skipping breakfast [15], another study, from the northern region of the country, stated that regular consumption of breakfast at home resulted in a normal BMI and a reduced likelihood of being underweight in male school children [35]. Further, a significant negative association between breakfast intake and BMI was observed in a large group of Saudi adolescents sampled from three major cities in the country [40]. However, a recent study involving male and female primary school students from Riyadh did not find any significant association between obesity levels and skipping breakfast [16]. Elsewhere, numerous studies from various countries have indicated that regular breakfast consumption is repeatedly associated with healthy body weight [7,8,13,14]. In addition, a systematic review conducted on the dietary correlates of obesity among children in the Middle East showed that several dietary behaviors, including skipping breakfast, were associated with obesity [41].

It is well recognized that the association between breakfast intake and obesity is confounded by many factors. Therefore, not all studies report a relationship between breakfast consumption and obesity. For instance, a recent cross-sectional study observed no association between breakfast consumption and children being overweight/obese [42]. Additionally, in a meta-analysis of observational studies, the cross-sectional studies showed that the risk of obesity in children and adolescents skipping breakfast was 43% greater than those who consumed breakfast regularly, while no significant association was found in cohort studies [43]. However, the number of cohort studies included in the meta-analysis was very small [43]. A recent review summarizing the relationship of skipping breakfast with body weight and metabolic outcomes in the child and adolescent population concluded that skipping breakfast was associated with overweight or obesity in 94.7% of the subjects [17]. Nonetheless, there were some heterogeneities in the definitions of overweight or obesity, skipping breakfast, and nutrient assessment, and confounding factors were infrequently reported [17]. This association between overweight/obesity, however, does not establish a causal relationship between them [44].

In the present study, a variety of foods were consumed by the Saudi children. Food choices made by children can be influenced by multiple factors, including family setting, friends, socioeconomic status, health considerations, food availability, color and taste, religious practices, and consumer trends. The findings showed that fried egg sandwiches, followed by breakfast cereals and spread cheese sandwiches were the foods most frequently consumed for breakfast, and those who consumed more cereals, labneh sandwiches, peanut butter sandwiches, and solid cheese sandwiches for breakfast were more likely to consume a daily breakfast. Some of the previous choices for breakfast were considered healthy choices, containing proteins and plenty of nutrients. A large body of epidemiological research has indicated that higher intake of ready-to-eat cereals (RTEC) by children is more likely to meet their recommended daily nutrient intake [45–47]. Indeed, RTEC consumption has been found to contribute to adequate key nutrient intake among children and adolescents in nationally representative cross-sectional data from the Canadian Community Health Survey (2015) [48]. The survey also showed that the nutrient density of the diet, as defined by the Nutrient-Rich Food Index, was significantly higher among RTEC consumers compared to non-consumers. In addition, RTEC consumption was not linked to overweight or obesity in this community study [48].

The study findings indicate that a higher percentage of boys (60.6%) than girls (46.8%) consumed fresh fruit at breakfast and that apples and bananas were the most consumed fruits with breakfast. A recent study from Riyadh, Saudi Arabia, reported contrasting findings to the ones found in the present study in relation to fruit consumption during breakfast, as girls consumed significantly more fresh fruit at breakfast than boys [16]. The present study showed that fruit intake in general was not associated with daily breakfast consumption. However, the Danish Health Behaviour in School-Aged Children Study (HBSC) reported that irregular breakfast consumption among adolescents was associated with a low frequency of fruit and vegetable consumption [49]. In addition, among Iranian school students aged 7 to 18 years, significant associations were found between skipping main meals, including breakfast, and low intake of fruits and vegetables [50].

Previous studies have shown that several factors can influence breakfast intake, including age, gender, family structure, and socio-economic status [12,19,37,51]. In the current study, there were no differences in breakfast intake due to age or gender. In agreement with the current findings, a recent study conducted on school children in Riyadh found similar results regarding breakfast consumption in relation to age or gender [16]. Findings from a Greek study showed that children of parents having more than 14 years of education were more likely to consume a daily breakfast [37]. Previous studies in various populations have reported a positive association between regular breakfast consumption and socioeconomic status [12,52,53]. In addition, there were a variety of familial-related factors that may influence breakfast consumption. Indeed, the family environment is considered an important influence on the dietary behaviors of children; therefore, family structure should be considered when designing programs to promote healthy breakfast habits [54]. In the current findings, mothers appeared to prepare breakfast most of the time, followed by domestic helpers. However, having domestic helpers prepare breakfast for the child appeared to associate with higher daily breakfast intake. A previous study conducted on Saudi children reported similar findings; mothers generally prepared breakfast at home, followed by domestic helpers. However, having breakfast prepared by a domestic helper was associated with non-daily breakfast consumption in that study [16].

The most prevalent reasons for not having regular breakfast at home in the present study included the child was not feeling hungry, the child waking up late with no time to have breakfast at home, and the child being given money to buy food from the school canteen. In another local study conducted on schoolgirls from Riyadh, the main reasons for not eating breakfast included not feeling hungry, not having enough time, or not having the preferred food choices available to them [15]. Needless to say, parents play an important role in children's eating behaviors through their attitudes and eating habits. In the present study, despite placing high importance (93.0%) on their children's breakfast intake, only 46% of the parents appeared satisfied with their children's breakfast intake. Those parents who considered breakfast to be a very important meal for their children were more likely to have their children consume daily breakfast. In a local study involving Saudi children from the central region of the country, parents also placed very high importance on breakfast compared to lunch or dinner [16].

Elsewhere, similar findings were reported by parents of elementary school-aged children in Bangkok, Thailand [39].

Unhealthy lifestyle behaviors were exhibited by a good proportion of children in the present study. Almost 70% of the children spend more than two hours of screen time daily, with boys being exceedingly spending more time on screen viewing than girls. Moreover, the majority of the children are considerably less active than the recommended daily time for physical activity, which is one hour of daily physical activity, with girls having significantly less physical activity than boys. Daily breakfast intake among school children was reported to be associated with a lower proportion of TV viewing time of more than two hours per day [25]. More screen time (more than two hours per day) increased the odds of skipping breakfast by almost 80% among Greek school children [38]. However, a study involving younger children from New Zealand aged 5 to 14 years found no association between breakfast intake and physical activity [55]. Findings from a multinational, cross-sectional study in 12 countries with 6228 children aged 9 to 11 years indicated that frequent breakfast consumption in the morning was related to a higher proportion of time spent in moderate to vigorous physical activity and a lower proportion of screen time compared with rare breakfast intake [56]. In a previous study conducted on Saudi adolescents, it was found that healthy versus unhealthy lifestyle habits cluster, as healthful dietary habits (intake of breakfast, fruits, vegetables, and milk) associate mostly with higher levels of physical activity, whereas unhealthful dietary habits (consumption of sugar-sweetened drinks, fast foods, cakes/donuts, and energy drinks) were related mostly to screen time [57].

It is well documented that adequate nocturnal sleep duration is an important part of maintaining good health and a sense of wellbeing among children and adolescents [58]. Two thirds of the sample in the present study did not have sufficient sleep duration at night (9 or more hours per night); however, more frequent breakfast intake was positively associated with sufficient nocturnal sleep among the current sample. A recent study conducted on children in Riyadh indicated that insufficient sleep duration was significantly associated with skipping daily breakfast [24]. More frequent intakes of breakfast were also reported to be significantly associated with adequate sleep duration among Saudi adolescents [59]. Indeed, the combination of insufficient sleep and skipping breakfast may have adverse effects on children's health. Numerous studies have reported a significant relationship between adequate sleep and daily breakfast intake. In a large group of Greek school children, insufficient sleep (<8 to 9 h per day) increased the odds of skipping breakfast by almost 80% [38]. Among a large number of Australian school children and adolescents, those who missed breakfast reported significantly poorer sleep [60]. Additionally, the proportion of Japanese adolescents who regularly consumed breakfast was significantly higher among those who slept for long durations [61]. In agreement with previously mentioned studies, adequate sleep among Taiwanese adolescents aged 13 to 18 years was related to eating a healthy diet, including having a daily breakfast [58].

Strengths and Limitations

The strengths of the present study include using a large and representative sample of Saudi children from both public and private schools in Jeddah. The study's analysis adjusted for important confounders, such as age, gender, and socioeconomic status. However, the present study has some limitations for consideration. First, the study has a cross-sectional design, which precludes us from inferring a causal relationship between breakfast intake and the selected variables. Second, the study did not exactly account for the cluster design effect. However, the size of the cluster was kept relatively small (nearly 16 students per class) and the sample size was further increased by 20% above the calculated one. Third, the breakfast intake and food choices were assessed using a questionnaire completed by the child's parents. Questionnaires are generally subject to recall bias and social desirability effects. Recall bias occurs when participants do not remember previous events or experiences accurately; however, asking the parent about routine or frequent events, such as information on typical breakfast intake of their children can minimize the recall bias to a great extent. Self-reporting bias represents an important problem in the assessment of most observational study, such as cross-sectional research. However, the anonymity of the respondent in the present study was an assuring factor to the parent. Fourth, although a clear definition of breakfast and adequate instructions were given to the parents, breakfast meaning can be subjectively interpreted by the respondents, as habitual breakfast is likely to vary among participants [62,63]. Fifth, Jeddah is a large cosmopolitan city with people from all parts of the country; however, the breakfast choices of the children in this city may not exactly reflect those of children living in rural areas of Saudi Arabia. Sixth, apart from the type of breakfast consumed, no further information on the quality and quantity of breakfast was assessed, as these two measures could be important in determining its health effects. Seventh, due to the large number of participants, we used a subjective assessment of physical activity rather than a more objective measure, such as motion sensors, which may have influenced the accuracy of the physical activity assessment. Therefore, the absolute physical activity levels presented in the current study should be interpreted with caution.

5. Conclusions

Skipping breakfast was found to be very prevalent among Saudi children, with no significant age or gender differences found. These findings corroborated earlier findings on breakfast consumption in other cities of the country. The most common reasons for not having breakfast at home included not being hungry and waking up late for school. Fried egg sandwiches, breakfast cereals, and spread cheese sandwiches were the foods most frequently consumed for breakfast. Strong parental support of breakfast as the main meal of the day was significantly associated with the more frequent breakfast intake in children. In addition, univariate analysis indicated that daily breakfast intake appears to associate significantly with the paternal and maternal education, getting sufficient nocturnal sleep, and having normal weight. However, logistic regression analysis adjusted for age, gender, and sociodemographic factors revealed that both paternal and maternal education, adequate sleep duration, and having BMI value lower than 25 kg/m^2 were all significantly associated with the more frequent breakfast intake in children.

The present findings have implications for children's health and school learning performance and indicate a need for concerted effort to promote daily breakfast consumption among Saudi school children. In addition, the findings of the present study in Jeddah, along with results from a similar study in Riyadh, which both show a high prevalence of skipping breakfast among Saudi children, raise a public health challenge. Prevention of breakfast skipping, increasing regular physical activity and reducing insufficient sleep and screen time can contribute to favorable lifestyle and dietary behaviors, as well as better overall health of Saudi children. Therefore, school children could be targeted for interventions to improve breakfast intake habits and overall lifestyle behaviors. Further, it is recommended that a nutrition education training for parents to be explored, in order to encourage and improve breakfast consumption habits among their school-age children.

Author Contributions: Conceptualization: H.M.A.-H., A.A.A.-R., L.J. and R.A.A.; methodology: H.M.A.-H., A.A.A.-R., L.J. and R.A.A.; investigation: H.M.A.-H., A.A.A.-R., L.J. and R.A.A.; data collection and supervision: A.A.A.-R., L.J. and R.A.A.; statistical analysis: H.M.A.-H.; interpretation of the findings: H.M.A.-H., A.A.A.-R., L.J. and R.A.A.; drafting the paper: H.M.A.-H.; reviewing and editing the draft: A.A.A.-R., L.J. and R.A.A.; funding acquisition: H.M.A.-H. All authors have read and agreed to the published version of the manuscript.

Funding: This research was supported by a grant from the Deanship of Scientific Research at Princess Nourah bint Abdulrahman University through the Fast-track Research Funding Program (Professor Hazzaa M. Al-Hazzaa).

Acknowledgments: We would like to thank all the participants for taking part in this study.

Conflicts of Interest: The authors declare that they have no competing interests.

References

1. Caprio, S.; Santoro, N.; Weiss, R. Childhood obesity and the associated rise in cardiometabolic complications. *Nat. Metab.* **2020**, *2*, 223–232. [CrossRef] [PubMed]
2. Simmonds, M.; Llewellyn, A.; Owen, C.; Woolacott, N. Predicting adult obesity from childhood obesity: A systematic review and meta-analysis. *Obes. Rev.* **2015**, *17*, 95–107.

3. Abarca-Gómez, L.; Abdeen, Z.A.; Hamid, Z.A.; Abu-Rmeileh, N.M.; Acosta-Cazares, B.; Acuin, C.; Adams, R.J.; Aekplakorn, W.; Afsana, K.; Aguilar-Salinas, C.A.; et al. Worldwide trends in body-mass index, underweight, overweight, and obesity from 1975 to 2016: A pooled analysis of 2416 population-based measurement studies in 128.9 million children, adolescents, and adults. *Lancet* **2017**, *390*, 2627–2642.
4. Al-Hussaini, A.A.; Bashir, M.S.; Khormi, M.; Alturaiki, M.; Alkhamis, W.; Alrajhi, M.; Halal, T. Overweight and obesity among Saudi children and adolescents: Where do we stand today? *Saudi J. Gastroenterol.* **2019**, *25*, 229–235. [PubMed]
5. Wen, L.M.; Rissel, C.; He, G. The effect of early life factors and early interventions on childhood overweight and obesity 2016. *J. Obes.* **2017**, *2017*, 3642818. [CrossRef]
6. Fang, J.; Gong, C.; Wan, Y.; Xu, Y.; Tao, F.; Sun, Y. Polygenic risk, adherence to a healthy lifestyle, and childhood obesity. *Pediatr. Obes.* **2019**, *14*, e12489. [CrossRef]
7. Blondin, S.; Anzman-Frasca, S.; Djang, H.; Economos, C. Breakfast consumption and adiposity among children and adolescents: An updated review of the literature. *Pediatr. Obes.* **2016**, *11*, 333–348.
8. Affenito, S.G.; Thompson, D.R.; Barton, B.A.; Franko, D.L.; Daniels, S.R.; Obarzanek, E.; Schreiber, G.B.; Striegel-Moore, R.H. Breakfast consumption by African-American and white adolescent girls correlates positively with calcium and fiber intake and negatively with body mass index. *J. Am. Diet. Assoc.* **2005**, *105*, 938–945.
9. Dubois, L.; Girard, M.; Potvin, K.M. Breakfast eating and overweight in a preschool population: Is there a link? *Public Health Nutr.* **2006**, *9*, 436–442.
10. Horikawa, C.; Kodama, S.; Yachi, Y.; Heianza, Y.; Hirasawa, R.; Ibe, Y.; Saito, K.; Shimano, H.; Yamada, N.; Sone, H.; et al. Skipping breakfast and prevalence of overweight and obesity in Asian and Pacific regions: A meta-analysis. *Prev. Med.* **2011**, *53*, 260–267. [PubMed]
11. Kyriazis, I.; Rekleiti, M.; Saridi, M.; Beliotis, E.; Toska, A.; Souliotis, K.; Wozniak, G. Prevalence of obesity in children aged 6–12 years in Greece: Nutritional behaviour and physical activity. *Arch. Med. Sci.* **2012**, *8*, 859–864. [CrossRef] [PubMed]
12. Timlin, M.T.; Pereira, M.A.; Story, M.; Neumark-Sztainer, D. Breakfast eating and weight change in a 5-year prospective analysis of adolescents: Project EAT (Eating Among Teens). *Pediatrics* **2008**, *121*, e638–e645. [CrossRef] [PubMed]
13. Yaguchi-Tanaka, Y.; Tabuchi, T. Skipping breakfast and subsequent overweight/obesity in children: A nationwide prospective study of 2.5 to 13-year olds in Japan. *J. Epidemiol.* **2020**. ahead of print. [CrossRef]
14. Sila, S.; Ilić, A.; Mišigoj-Duraković, M.; Sorić, M.; Radman, I.; Šatalić, Z. Obesity in adolescents who skip breakfast is not associated with physical activity. *Nutrients* **2019**, *11*, 2511. [CrossRef]
15. Al Turki, M.; Al Shloi, S.; Al Harbi, A.; Al Agil, A.; Philip, W.; Qureshi, S. Breakfast consumption habits among schoolchildren: A cross-sectional study in Riyadh, Saudi Arabia. *Int. Res. J. Med. Med. Sci.* **2018**, *6*, 50–55.
16. Al-Hazzaa, H.M.; Alhowikan, A.M.; Alhussain, M.H.; Obeid, O.A. Breakfast consumption among Saudi primary-school children relative to sex and socio-demographic factors. *BMC Public Health* **2020**, *20*, 448. [CrossRef]
17. Monzani, A.; Ricotti, R.; Caputo, M.; Solito, A.; Archero, F.; Bellone, S.; Prodam, F. A systematic review of the association of skipping breakfast with weight and cardiometabolic risk factors in children and adolescents. What should we better investigate in the future? *Nutrients* **2019**, *11*, 387. [CrossRef]
18. Adolphus, K.; Lawton, C.L.; Dye, L. The effects of breakfast on behavior and academic performance in children and adolescents. *Front. Hum. Neurosci.* **2013**, *7*, 425.
19. Rampersaud, G.C.; Pereira, M.A.; Girard, B.L.; Adams, J.; Metzl, J.D. Breakfast habits, nutritional status, body weight, and academic performance in children and adolescents. *J. Am. Diet. Assoc.* **2005**, *105*, 743–760. [PubMed]
20. Widenhorn-Müller, K.; Hille, K.; Klenk, J.; Weiland, U. Influence of having breakfast on cognitive performance and mood in 13-to 20-year-old high school students: Results of a crossover trial. *Pediatrics* **2008**, *122*, 279–284.
21. Mielgo-Ayuso, J.; Valtueña, J.; Cuenca-García, M.; Gottrand, F.; Breidenassel, C.; Ferrari, M.; Manios, Y.; De Henauw, S.; Widhalm, K.; Kafatos, A.; et al. Regular breakfast consumption is associated with higher blood vitamin status in adolescents: The HELENA (healthy lifestyle in Europe by nutrition in adolescence) study. *Public Health Nutr.* **2017**, *20*, 1393–1404. [CrossRef] [PubMed]

22. Ramsay, S.A.; Bloch, T.D.; Marriage, B.; Shriver, L.H.; Spees, C.K.; Taylor, C.A. Skipping breakfast is associated with lower diet quality in young US children. *Eur. J. Clin. Nutr.* **2018**, *72*, 548–556. [CrossRef] [PubMed]
23. Mounayar, R.; Jreij, R.; Hachem, J.; Abboud, F.; Tueni, M. Breakfast intake and factors associated with adherence to the Mediterranean diet among Lebanese high school adolescents. *J. Nutr. Metab.* **2019**, *2019*, 2714286. [CrossRef] [PubMed]
24. Al-Hazzaa, H.M.; Alhussain, M.H.; Alhowikan, A.M.; Obeid, O.A. Insufficient sleep duration and its association with breakfast intake, overweight/obesity, socio-demographics and selected lifestyle behaviors among Saudi school children. *Nat. Sci. Sleep* **2019**, *11*, 253–263. [CrossRef]
25. Vereecken, C.; The HBSC Eating & Dieting Focus Group; Dupuy, M.; Rasmussen, M.; Kelly, C.; Nansel, T.R.; Al Sabbah, H.; Baldassari, D.; Jordan, M.D.; Maes, L.; et al. Breakfast consumption and its socio-demographic and lifestyle correlates in schoolchildren in 41 countries participating in the HBSC study. *Int. J. Public Health* **2009**, *54* (Suppl. 2), 180–190. [CrossRef]
26. Al-Othaimeen, A.; Osman, A.K.; Al Orf, S. Prevalence of nutritional anaemia among primary school girls in Riyadh City, Saudi Arabia. *Int. J. Food Sci. Nutr.* **1999**, *50*, 237–243. [CrossRef]
27. Abalkhail, B.; Shawky, S. Prevalence of daily breakfast intake, iron deficiency anaemia and awareness of being anaemic among Saudi school students. *Int. J. Food Sci. Nutr.* **2002**, *53*, 519–528. [CrossRef]
28. AL-Oboudi, L.M. Impact of breakfast eating pattern on nutritional status, glucose level, iron status in blood and test grades among upper primary school girls in Riyadh city, Saudi Arabia. *Pakistan J. Nutr.* **2010**, *9*, 106–111. Available online: http://citeseerx.ist.psu.edu/viewdoc/download?doi=10.1.1.624.9904&rep=rep1&type=pdf (accessed on 25 May 2020). [CrossRef]
29. Cole, T.J.; Lobstein, T. Extended International (IOTF) body mass index cut-offs for thinness, overweight and obesity. *Pediatr. Obes.* **2012**, *7*, 284–294. [CrossRef]
30. American Academy of Pediatrics. Committee on Public Education. American academy of pediatrics: Children, adolescents, and television. *Pediatrics* **2001**, *107*, 423–426. [CrossRef]
31. Canadian Society for Exercise Physiology. Canadian 24-Hour Movement Guidelines for Children and Youth (Ages 5–17 Years). 2020. Available online: https://csepguidelines.ca/children-and-youth-5-17/ (accessed on 15 October 2020).
32. Hirshkowitz, M.; Whiton, K.; Albert, S.M.; Alessi, C.; Bruni, O.; DonCarlos, L.; Hazen, N.; Herman, J.; Katz, E.S. National Sleep Foundation's sleep time duration recommendations: Methodology and results summary. *Sleep Health* **2015**, *1*, 40–43. [CrossRef] [PubMed]
33. Tremblay, M.S.; Warburton, D.E.; Janssen, I.; Paterson, D.H.; Latimer, A.E.; Rhodes, R.E.; Kho, M.E.; Hicks, A.; Leblanc, A.G.; Zehr, L.; et al. New Canadian physical activity guidelines. *Appl. Physiol. Nutr. Metab.* **2011**, *36*, 47–58. [CrossRef]
34. Farghaly, N.F.; Ghazali, B.M.; Al-Wabel, H.M.; Sadek, A.A.; Abbag, F.I. Life style and nutrition and their impact on health of Saudi school students in Abha, Southwestern region of Saudi Arabia. *Saudi Med. J.* **2007**, *28*, 415–421. [PubMed]
35. Alenazi, S.A.; Ali, H.W.; Alshammary, O.M.; Alenazi, M.S.; Wazir, F. Effect of breakfast on body mass index (BMI) in male children in northern border region Saudi Arabia. *Khyber Med. Univ. J.* **2014**, *6*, 106–109.
36. Smith, K.J.; Breslin, M.C.; McNaughton, S.A.; Gall, S.L.; Blizzard, L.; Venn, A.J. Skipping breakfast among Australian children and adolescents; findings from the 2011–2012 National Nutrition and Physical Activity Survey. *Aust. N. Z. J. Public Health* **2017**, *41*, 572–578. [CrossRef]
37. Manios, Y.; Moschonis, G.; Androutsos, O.; Filippou, C.; Van Lippevelde, W.; Vik, F.N.; Velde, S.J.T.; Jan, N.; Dössegger, A.; Bere, E.; et al. Family sociodemographic characteristics as correlates of children's breakfast habits and weight status in eight European countries. The ENERGY (EuropeaN Energy balance research to prevent excessive weight gain among youth) project. *Public Health Nutr.* **2015**, *18*, 774–783. [CrossRef]
38. Tambalis, K.D.; Panagiotakos, D.B.; Psarra, G.; Sidossis, L.S. Breakfast skipping in Greek schoolchildren connected to an unhealthy lifestyle profile. Results from the National Action for Children's Health program. *Nutr. Diet* **2019**, *76*, 328–335. [CrossRef]
39. Sirichakwal, P.P.; Janesiripanich, N.; Kunapun, P.; Senaprom, S.; Purttipornthanee, S. Breakfast consumption behaviors of elementary school children in Bangkok metropolitan region. *Southeast Asian J. Trop. Med. Public Health* **2015**, *46*, 939–948.

40. Al-Hazzaa, H.M.; Abahussain, N.; Al-Sobayel, H.; Qahwaji, D.; Musaiger, A.O. Physical activity, sedentary behaviors and dietary habits among Saudi adolescents relative to age, gender and region. *Int. J. Behav. Nutr. Phys. Act.* **2011**, *8*, 140. [CrossRef]
41. Albataineh, S.R.; Badran, E.F.; Tayyem, R.F. Dietary factors and their association with childhood obesity in the Middle East: A systematic review. *Nutr. Health* **2019**, *25*, 53–60. [CrossRef]
42. Champilomati, G.; Notara, V.; Prapas, C.; Konstantinou, E.; Kordoni, M.; Velentza, A.; Mesimeri, M.; Antonogeorgos, G.; Rojas-Gil, A.P.; Kornilaki, E.N.; et al. Breakfast consumption and obesity among preadolescents: An epidemiological study. *Pediatr. Int.* **2020**, *62*, 81–88. [CrossRef] [PubMed]
43. Ardeshirlarijani, E.; Namazi, N.; Jabbari, M.; Zeinali, M.; Gerami, H.; Jalili, R.B.; Larijani, B.; Azadbakht, L. The link between breakfast skipping and overweigh/obesity in children and adolescents: A meta-analysis of observational studies. *J. Diabetes Metab. Disord.* **2019**, *18*, 657–664. [CrossRef] [PubMed]
44. Brown, A.W.; Brown, M.M.; Allison, D.B. Belief beyond the evidence: Using the proposed effect of breakfast on obesity to show 2 practices that distort scientific evidence. *Am. J. Clin. Nutr.* **2013**, *98*, 1298–1308. [CrossRef] [PubMed]
45. Albertson, A.M.; Affenito, S.G.; Bauserman, R.; Holschuh, N.M.; Eldridge, A.L.; Barton, B.A. The relationship of ready-to-eat cereal consumption to nutrient intake, blood lipids, and body mass index of children as they age through adolescence. *J. Am. Diet. Assoc.* **2009**, *109*, 1557–1565. [CrossRef]
46. Van den Boom, A.; Serra-Majem, L.; Ribas, L.; Ngo, J.; Pérez-Rodrigo, C.; Aranceta, J.; Fletcher, R. The contribution of ready-to-eat cereals to daily nutrient intake and breakfast quality in a Mediterranean setting. *J. Am. Coll. Nutr.* **2006**, *25*, 135–143. [CrossRef]
47. Williams, P.G. The benefits of breakfast cereal consumption: A systematic review of the evidence base. *Adv. Nutr.* **2014**, *5*, 636S–673S. [CrossRef]
48. Vatanparast, H.; Islam, N.; Patil, R.P.; Shamloo, A.; Keshavarz, P.; Smith, J.; Chu, L.M.; Whiting, S. Consumption of Ready-to-Eat Cereal in Canada and its contribution to nutrient intake and nutrient density among Canadians. *Nutrients* **2019**, *11*, 1009. [CrossRef]
49. Pedersen, T.P.; Meilstrup, C.; Holstein, B.E.; Rasmussen, M. Fruit and vegetable intake is associated with frequency of breakfast, lunch and evening meal: Cross-sectional study of 11-, 13-, and 15-year-olds. *Int. J. Behav. Nutr. Phys. Act.* **2012**, *9*, 9. [CrossRef]
50. Pourrostami, K.; Heshmat, R.; Hemati, Z.; Heidari-Beni, M.; Qorbani, M.; Motlagh, M.E.; Raeisi, A.; Shafiee, G.; Ziaodini, H.; Beshtar, S.; et al. Association of fruit and vegetable intake with meal skipping in children and adolescents: The CASPIAN-V study. *Eat. Weight Disord.* **2019**, *25*, 903–910. [CrossRef]
51. Levin, K.; Kirby, J.; Currie, C. Family structure and breakfast consumption of 11–15 year old boys and girls in Scotland, 1994–2010: A repeated cross-sectional study. *BMC Public Health* **2012**, *12*, 228. [CrossRef]
52. Johansen, A.; Rasmussen, S.; Madsen, M. Health behaviour among adolescents in Denmark: Influence of school class and individual risk factors. *Scand. J. Public Health* **2006**, *34*, 32–40. [CrossRef] [PubMed]
53. Keski-Rahkonen, A.; Kaprio, J.; Rissanen, A.; Virkkunen, M.; Rose, R.J. Breakfast skipping and health-compromising behaviors in adolescents and adults. *Eur. J. Clin. Nutr.* **2003**, *57*, 842–853. [CrossRef] [PubMed]
54. Pearson, N.; Biddle, S.J.; Gorely, T. Family correlates of breakfast consumption among children and adolescents. A systematic review. *Appetite* **2009**, *52*, 1–7. [CrossRef] [PubMed]
55. Utter, J.; Scragg, R.; Mhurchu, C.N.; Schaaf, D. At-home breakfast consumption among New Zealand children: Associations with body mass index and related nutrition behaviors. *J. Am. Diet. Assoc.* **2007**, *107*, 570–576. [CrossRef]
56. Zakrzewski-Fruer, J.K.; Gillison, F.B.; Katzmarzyk, P.T.; Mire, E.F.; Broyles, S.T.; Champagne, C.M.; Chaput, J.-P.; Denstel, K.D.; Fogelholm, M.; Gang, H.; et al. Association between breakfast frequency and physical activity and sedentary time: A cross-sectional study in children from 12 countries. *BMC Public Health* **2019**, *19*, 222. [CrossRef]
57. Al-Hazzaa, H.M.; Al-Sobayel, H.I.; Abahussain, N.A.; Qahwaji, D.M.; Alahmadi, M.A.; Musaiger, A.O. Association of dietary habits with levels of physical activity and screen time among adolescents living in Saudi Arabia. *J. Hum. Nutr. Diet.* **2014**, *27* (Suppl. 2), 204–213. [CrossRef]
58. Chen, M.-Y.; Wang, E.K.; Jeng, Y.-J. Adequate sleep among adolescents is positively associated with health status and health-related behaviors. *BMC Public Health* **2006**, *6*, 59. [CrossRef]

59. Al-Hazzaa, H.M.; Musaiger, A.O.; Abahussain, N.A.; Al-Sobayel, H.I.; Qahwaji, D.M. Lifestyle correlates of self-reported sleep duration among Saudi adolescents: A multicentre school-based cross-sectional study. *Child. Care Health Dev.* **2014**, *40*, 533–542. [CrossRef]
60. Agostini, A.; Lushington, K.; Kohler, M.; Dorrian, J. Associations between self-reported sleep measures and dietary behaviours in a large sample of Australian school students ($n = 28{,}010$). *J. Sleep Res.* **2018**, *27*, e12682. [CrossRef]
61. Tanaka, H.; Taira, K.; Arakawa, M.; Masuda, A.; Yamamoto, Y.; Komoda, Y.; Kadegaru, H.; Shirakawa, S. An examination of sleep health, lifestyle and mental health in junior high school students. *Psychiatry Clin. Neurosci.* **2002**, *56*, 235–236. [CrossRef]
62. Adolphus, K.; Bellissimo, N.; Lawton, C.L.; Ford, N.A.; Rains, T.M.; de Zepetnek, J.T.; Dye, L. Methodological challenges in studies examining the effects of breakfast on cognitive performance and appetite in children and adolescents. *Adv. Nutr.* **2017**, *8*, 184S–196S. [CrossRef] [PubMed]
63. O'Neil, C.E.; Byrd-Bredbenner, C.; Hayes, D.; Jana, L.; Klinger, S.E.; Stephenson-Martin, S. The role of breakfast in health: Definition and criteria for a quality breakfast. *J. Acad. Nutr. Diet.* **2014**, *114* (Suppl. 12), S8–S26. [CrossRef] [PubMed]

Publisher's Note: MDPI stays neutral with regard to jurisdictional claims in published maps and institutional affiliations.

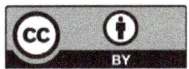

© 2020 by the authors. Licensee MDPI, Basel, Switzerland. This article is an open access article distributed under the terms and conditions of the Creative Commons Attribution (CC BY) license (http://creativecommons.org/licenses/by/4.0/).

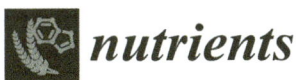

Article

A Cross-Sectional Survey of Salty Snack Consumption among Serbian Urban-Living Students and Their Contribution to Salt Intake

Jasmina B. Timic [1,*], Jelena Kotur-Stevuljevic [2], Heiner Boeing [3], Dušanka Krajnovic [4], Brizita Djordjevic [1] and Sladjana Sobajic [1]

1. Department of Bromatology, Faculty of Pharmacy, University of Belgrade, Vojvode Stepe 450, 11221 Belgrade, Serbia; brizitadjordjevic@gmail.com (B.D.); sladjana.sobajic@pharmacy.bg.ac.rs (S.S.)
2. Department of Medical Biochemistry, Faculty of Pharmacy, University of Belgrade, Vojvode Stepe 450, 11221 Belgrade, Serbia; jkotur@pharmacy.bg.ac.rs
3. Data Analysis Unit, National Institute of Gastroenterology "Saverio de Bellis", Research Hospital, Castellana Grotte, 70013 Bari, Italy; boeing@dife.de
4. Department of Social Pharmacy and Pharmaceutical Legislation, Faculty of Pharmacy, University of Belgrade, Vojvode Stepe 450, 11221 Belgrade, Serbia; dusica.krajnovic@pharmacy.bg.ac.rs
* Correspondence: jassminatimic@gmail.com; Tel.: +381-11-3951-326

Received: 14 September 2020; Accepted: 21 October 2020; Published: 27 October 2020

Abstract: This study investigated the behavior of urban-living students related to the salty snacks consumption, and their contribution to salt daily intake. A cross-sectional survey on 1313 urban-living students (16–25 years, 61.4% university students and 38.6% high school students) used a pre-verified questionnaire created specifically for the study. The logistic regression analysis was performed to investigate the factors influencing snack consumption. The results of salt content and the snack consumption frequency were used to evaluate snack contribution to salt intake. All subjects consumed salty snacks, on average several times per week, more often at home and slightly more during periods of intensive studying, with 42% of the participants reporting to consume two or more packages per snacking occasion. Most of the participants consumed such products between main meals, but 10% of them took snacks immediately after the main meal. More high-school students than university students were in the "high snack group" ($p < 0.05$). The most frequently consumed salty snacks were those with the highest content of salt. Salt intake from snack products for a majority of participants ranged between 0.4 and 1 g/day. The research revealed younger age, home environment and significant contribution to salt intake as critical points in salty snack consumption among urban-living students important for the better understanding of their dietary habits.

Keywords: salty snack products; students; consumption; salt intake

---

1. Introduction

Adolescence is an important period in life in which food choices are starting to become individually settled. Some food choices such as skipping meals, irregular meals, a low consumption of fruits and vegetables, often snacking on high-energy-dense foods, and drinking high-energy-dense beverages, are considered detrimental to health in the long-term [1]. Snacking among children and adolescents has become very common worldwide, with an increase of over 20% on a daily basis over the past 30 years [2]. The attitudes and habits associated with snacking and snack product consumption in the population of young people have been investigated in many countries in recent years [3–6]. Snacking trends among children in the United States (USA) in the period between 1989 and 2006 saw an enormous increase, with an average of three snacks per day, and more than 27% of daily calories coming from snacks. The highest increases were associated with salty snacks and candies. Over 24% of adolescents in Mexico consumed salty snacks every day [4], whereas young adults aged 16–24 years in United Kingdom consumed snacks more than 2.5 times a day [6]. Apart from the snack consumption frequency and demographic characteristics, it was of interest to study the correlation between snacking and the body mass index, social, economic, and psychological determinants, and the influence of the environment and circumstances on snacking patterns [7,8].

Generally speaking, snack food is a broad term covering a heterogeneous, wide, and diverse range of products, coming in a variety of forms, including pre-packaged snack foods and food items made at home. Most of the studies considered snack foods to be one product group [3,9,10] while researchers less frequently conducted studies that addressed one particular snack type. Salty snacks differ in their composition from other snack products, especially in terms of salt and sugar content [11]. In addition, not much is known to what extent salty snacks contribute to salt intake. The salt content in these food items may be high contributing to an excessive intake of sodium, which is associated with high blood pressure and adverse cardiovascular events. In one of the rare studies of this kind Ponzo et al. [12] have found that almost half of the average daily sodium intake in Italian adolescents originated from salty snacks and that their blood pressure was positively correlated with the frequency of salty snack consumption.

The World Health Organization's framework "Shake the Salt Habit" emphasizes the importance of identifying the salt dietary sources in order to better formulate salt reduction strategies [13]. Since no previous study of salty snack intake among young people had been conducted in Serbia, the present study investigated high-school and university students from urban areas for the purpose of examining their habits of consuming salty snacks and their importance as salt dietary sources in this population. Our specific objective was to find out whether there are age-related and behavioral differences in the consumption of salty snack products and to identify the factors which contribute to their being high consumers. These kinds of data are also important for developing future educational programs for salt reduction intake and for potential product reformulation options.

2. Materials and Methods

2.1. Study Population

The final study population included 1313 students from an urban area. The participants were recruited from two public high schools types ($N = 507$; medical school and gymnasium) and two state faculties ($N = 806$; study areas pharmacy and management/organization) in order to portray the attitudes and habits of urban-living young people of different educational background. The schools and faculties were located in the central area of Belgrade, capitol of Serbia, high-school size was >300, and faculty size was >1000 students. Participation was completely voluntary without incentives and required no registration of personal data. The inclusion criterion was age (14–19 for high-school students and 18–27 for university students). The exclusion criterion was the lack of inclusion criteria. Data collection was conducted during 2016 and 2017. The study itself was approved by the Ethics Committee for Biomedical Research of the Faculty of Pharmacy, University of Belgrade, Republic of Serbia (project identification code 164/3, date of approval 25 February 2015).

2.2. Questionnaires

Lifestyle and dietary habit questionnaire was compiled specifically for the study and was pre-tested on 30 students prior to the examination to determine the time needed for completion and the level of understanding. The internal consistency of its questions was tested using Cronbach's α. The survey included 12 brief questions that were divided into several topics and a food frequency questionnaire (FFQ). The participants were asked to fill out the questionnaire in one session in the classroom environment at schools or during breaks between lectures at faculties. All questionnaires were coded with 4-letter codes randomly chosen by the participants. The topics covered by the questionnaire were as follows: demographic characteristics, body weight and height, education level, overall dietary habits, participants' perception of their diet quality, and their habits related to consuming salty snack products. The self-reported weight and height data of the participants were used to calculate the body mass index (BMI) and further classification of nutritional status was based on the World Health Organization (WHO) criteria [14]. A structured FFQ was additional part of lifestyle and habit questionnaire and was used to collect information about the frequency of salty snack intake (FFQ). In the FFQ, snack products were grouped into categories and included popular salty snack products available on the market, such as chips, flips, popcorn, fried corn, salted sticks, pretzels, crackers, fish-shaped products, roasted and baked nuts, seeds, and salted peanuts. It was also possible to include additional products.

A 72-h dietary recall questionnaire (DR1) on salty snack consumption was conducted on all the participants concurrently with the lifestyle questionnaire, and again 2 months later on 15% of the formerly surveyed population (100 university and 100 high-school students, total $N = 200$). This second survey was not announced in advance and the inclusion criteria were previous engagement in the study and the availability to give answers to DR2 survey (only students that were available and willing at this second occasion participated in DR2). Gender and age characteristics of this sub-group reflected the same characteristics of all participating students. This sub-group of participants was asked to self-code DR2 with the same 4-letter codes as previously. Information about the product type and brand, and the weight and number of packages consumed in last 72 h was collected in DR1 and DR2. The results from DR1 and DR2 for 6 days in total were used to calculate quantitative salt intake (see below).

2.3. Salt Content of Snacks

The salt content analysis was carried out employing the Association of Official Analytical Chemists (AOAC) official titrimetric method 950.52 [15]. An internal method control was conducted on a weekly basis using the laboratory chloride standard and samples fortified at 3 concentration levels. A total of 122 samples that included 48 different salty pre-packaged food products were purchased from supermarkets, local shops, and health food stores. The number of samples from different lots that were analyzed ranged between 1 and 7.

2.4. Assessment of Chronic Salt Exposure

The results from DR1 and DR2 for 6 days in total for the same sub-group of participants ($N = 200$, confirmed with the match in codes) were used to calculate quantitative salt intake. The observed individual means (OIM) model within the Monte Carlo risk assessment method (MCRA) was employed [16]. In the OIM approach, chronic exposure was calculated using information about salt content in different salty snack products (results obtained from a chemical analysis in our laboratory) and the product type and quantity consumed over the previous 72 h for 200 participants (DR1 and DR2, in total 6 days). Average exposures to salt from salty snack products per participant/day were calculated as follows: each salty snack product consumed by a single participant was multiplied with the mean salt concentration in that product. Exposures from products consumed during 6 recorded days were summed up to obtain the average daily exposure for that person.

2.5. Statistical Analysis

Statistical data processing was performed employing Predictive Analytics SoftWare (PASW SPSS), version 18 (Chicago, IL, USA). ANOVA test (with post-hoc Tukey test) for continuous variables comparison, while Chi-square tests for discrete variables were applied to verify the possible differences in sub-groups according to different criteria. For 2 × 2 contingency tables Fisher exact test with Yates correction testing difference in frequencies in distinct categories were implemented.

The logistic regression analysis was performed in order to assess different factors which determined the number of snacks regularly consumed by the subjects of the present study. From the logistic regression models, odds ratios (ORs) were estimated with their corresponding 95% confidence intervals. A p value < 0.05 was considered as statistically significant.

Regarding reliability testing of the FFQ's internal consistency Cronbach's α coefficient analysis was used. Test–retest analysis was obtained as a correlation analysis between questionnaire's items in two time points. Exploratory factorial analysis of the questionnaire was made in order to get classified main factors by using principal component analysis as extraction method. Variance value of each factor was measured by distinct eigen value. Factorial analysis validity was tested by the Kaiser–Meyer–Olkin measure of sampling adequacy and Bartlett's test of sphericity. Rotation was performed with Varimax method. The main characteristic of the extracted factors was percentage of variance explained. Extracted factors were entitled according to items nature and meaning.

3. Results

The research covered 1313 respondents, of whom 72.4% were females and 27.6% males. The study population included 806 students from faculties (61.4%) and 507 students from high-schools (38.6%). The respondents' age ranged from 16 to 25 years. The mean age among students was 23 years and among high-school students 17 years. On average, the mean BMI for university students was 21 ± 2.7 kg/m^2 and 21 ± 2.5 kg/m^2 for high-school students. Supplementary Table S1 features the descriptive characteristics of the population.

Cronbach's alpha of the questionnaire was 0.865, which is rated as very good reliability. No questionnaire item deleted value was larger than basic value of 0.865, so it could be concluded that all questions were consistent with the questionnaire topic. The interclass correlation coefficient (single measures) was 0.368 (95% confidence interval 0.244–0.535; F = 9.409, df1 = 29, df2 = 2290, $p < 0.001$). Average inter-item correlation coefficient was 0.365 ± 0.039 which suggested relatively strong correlation between items (the average correlation coefficient is acceptable if it is larger than 0.300). Test–retest analysis showed good correlation between different items in two time points (average Spearman's $\varrho = 0.785$; $p < 0.01$). Principal component analysis method was used for factorial analysis. The Kaiser–Meyer–Olkin parameter for sampling adequacy was 0.608 and the Bartlett's test of sphericity was statistically significant ($p < 0.001$). Using Varimax rotation four factors were extracted, explaining in total 74.6% of variance. The first factor was related to the main pattern of salty snack consumption (items: dominant place of consumption, frequency of consumption, time of consumption regarding the main meal, and product type) and carried 35.2%; the second that described information influence on snack eating habits (awareness of nutritive value) carried 17,3%; the third 12.3%, and was related to the general dietary habits (items: number of main meals, number of refreshments, eating with nonalcoholic or alcoholic beverages, and eating in front of TV); and the fourth was on personal preferences (university/high school, motivational reasons for consumption, and day period related consumption) carried 9.9% of variance (Supplementary Table S2).

As far as the school food environment is concerned, no canteens were available at high schools, but canteens were available for students at their faculties. Vending machines of different types dispensing snacks and beverages were provided on school and faculty premises.

All of the participating students self-reported consuming salty snacks. Serbian youngsters cited "bakery products" (salted sticks, fish-shaped products, pretzels, and bake rolls) as the most popular type of snack products. The next most popularly consumed snacks were chips and popcorn, followed by peanuts, nuts and seeds, flips, and crackers.

The frequency of salty snack consumption, and the number and size of packages consumed were ascertained in the FFQ (Table 1). More than 90% of all the respondents reported eating snack products from several times per month to several times per week. Some 7% of them consumed salty snack products every day, whereas as few as 2.3% reported eating salty snack products most commonly several times a day. Comparing the frequency of snack product intake, substantially different habits were observed among the selected groups. More specifically, the pupil group showed a higher tendency to a more frequent intake of snack products (statistically significant "once per week" and "several times per day"; $p < 0.05$). The results pertaining to the number of packages and time of day when salty snack products were most commonly consumed are featured in Table 1. Concerning the number of packages of salty snack products usually consumed during one snacking occasion, results showed that 37.2% university and 49.3% high-school students regularly consumed multiple packages. More university students than high-school students consumed these products at home (70% and 54%, respectively), while more high-school than university students consumed the same type of snacks at school (34% and 17%, respectively) (Table 1). In terms of the vicinity of the main meals when participants usually consumed salty snack products, the most common answers were "between the main meals" and "immediately after the main meal". Substantially more high-school students reported that they often take snack products immediately after the main meal and between the main meals as compared to university students ($p < 0.001$), whereas more university students consumed salty snacks instead of the main meal. However, the intake of snacks instead of, before or during the main meal, remained at a very low level. More than one-half of the respondents reported that they sometimes eat snacks in front of the TV set/computer and more than 30% tend to do so very often. The most preferable part of day for salty snack consumption was evening in both groups of students.

Table 1. Characteristics of salty snack consumption among students.

Frequency of Snack Consumption	All	High-School Student	University Student
1–3 times per month	394 (30.0%)	141 (27.9%)	253 (31.4%)
Once per week	397 (30.2%)	135 (26.7%)	262 (32.5%) *
2–3 times per week	404 (30.8%)	169 (33.4%)	235 (29.1%)
Daily	88 (6.7%)	42 (8.3%)	46 (5.7%)
Several times per day	30 (2.3%)	19 (3.8%)	11 (1.4%) **
	$\chi^2, p *$ 17.2, <0.01		
Place of usual snack consumption			
At home	819 (62.4%)	262 (51.8%)	557 (69.0%) ***
At school/university	302 (23.0%)	163 (32.2%)	98 (17.2%) ***
Out-of-doors	157 (12.0%)	59 (11.7%)	98 (12.2%)
Other	35 (2.6%)	22 (4.3%)	13 (1.6%) **
	$\chi^2, p *$ 46.7, <0.001		
Snack consumption in front of the TV or computer			
Often	448 (34.1%)	157 (30.8%)	292 (36.2%)
Sometimes	698 (53.2%)	279 (55.1%)	418 (51.7%)
Never	167 (12.7%)	70 (13.8%)	97 (12.0%)
	$\chi^2, p *$ 5.7, NS		
Number of snack packages			
One package	763 (58.1%)	256 (50.7%)	507 (62.8%) ***
Two packages	355 (27.0%)	155 (30.6%)	200 (24.8%) *
Three packages	135 (10.3%)	61 (12.1%)	74 (9.2%)
Four packages and more	60 (4.6%)	34 (6.7%)	26 (3.2%) **
	$\chi^2, p *$ 26.1, <0.001		
Snack consumption time			
Before the main meal	27 (2.1%)	10 (2.0%)	17 (2.1%)
During the main meal	4 (0.3%)	1 (0.2%)	3 (0.4%)
Immediately after the main meal	116 (8.8%)	55 (10.9%)	61 (7.6%)
Between the main meals	814 (62%)	371 (73.3%)	443 (54.9%) ***
Instead of the main meal	22 (1.7%)	3 (0.6%)	19 (2.4%) *
Other	330 (25.1%)	264 (32.7%)	66 (13.0%) ***
	$\chi^2, p *$ 103.4, <0.001		

χ^2, p = from the Chi square test comparing pupils and students' sub-groups; *, **, *** $p < 0.05, 0.01$, and 0.001, respectively. Fisher exact test with Yates correction testing difference in frequencies in distinct categories. NS = not significant. The study groups were further divided according to the daily number of snack products consumed into the "low group" (once to several times per month), "medium group" (two to four times per week) and "high group" (once or several times per day). BMI did not differ between snack frequency subgroups, while high-school/university student ratio was significantly different. The majority of students (>50%) belonged to the "low group", followed by almost one third of students in the "medium group". Higher percent of university students belonged to the low intake group compared to the percent of high-school students, which suggested that younger students were more prone to frequently use salty snack products (Table 2).

Table 2. Frequency of salty snack product consumption based on students' age and weight status.

Parameter	Low Snack Intake N = 791	Medium Snack Intake N = 404	High Snack Intake N = 118	p
Age, years	21.5 ± 3.4	23.1 ± 2.1 aaa	20.3 ± 2.7 aaa, bbb	<0.001
BMI kg/m^2	21.2 ± 2.7	20.8 ± 2.4	21.0 ± 2.9	0.157
<25 kg/m^2	727 (59.7%)	384 (31.6%)	106 (8.7%)	χ^2 = 5.4; 0.065
25–30	64 (66.7%)	20 (20.8%)	12 (12.5%)	
High-school students (n = 507)	276 (54.5%)	169 (33.4%)	61 (12.1%)	χ^2 = 14.9; 0.001
University students (n = 806)	515 (63.8%)	235 (29.1%)	57 (7.1%)	

ANOVA test with post-hoc Tukey test is used for continuous variables comparison: age and BMI. aaa, bbb $p < 0.001$ vs. low snack and medium snack intake groups, respectively. Chi-square test is used for categorical variables. BMI, body mass index.

The binary logistic regression analysis was performed to assess the factors which contributed to being a high snack consumer (once or more times per day) in comparison with the low group among all subjects of this study and also in high-school/university student subgroups. Statistical significance was taken into account for $p < 0.05$. Resulted significance values (p-values) of this part of analyses are presented in Table 3, while in Supplementary Table S3 a comprehensive statistical data are shown.

Table 3. Logistic regression analysis of the variables (questionnaire's items) that could predict a high level of salty snack product intake among the population of urban living students.

Population	All	High-School Students	University Students
	p	p	p
Gender m/f	0.943	0.401	0.537
Age (years)	<0.001	<0.01	0.378
BMI	0.515	0.464	0.834
Type of snack products	<0.001	<0.001	<0.001
Awareness of SP nutritive value	<0.05	0.540	<0.05
Morning consumption	<0.001	<0.001	<0.01
Midday consumption	<0.001	<0.001	<0.001
Evening consumption	<0.001	<0.001	<0.001
Motivation reasons	0.187	0.245	0.932
Number of main meals	0.117	0.271	0.436
Number of refreshments	<0.001	<0.001	<0.01
Self-perception of overall diet quality	<0.001	<0.001	0.182

p-values present significance level of distinct factors for high snack usage prediction; SP-salty snack product; m/f—male/female.

Performing the same analysis in separate high-school and university student groups, we revealed that among high-school students the most important predictors of salty snack usage quantity were all three day-period related frequencies, number of refreshments, and self-perception towards diet quality, while in an university student group these factors were midday and evening consumption frequency only. The most important variables (items) that determined the high frequency of salty snack products consumption for all participants together included age, snack type, morning, midday and evening consumption frequency, number of refreshments, and self-perception towards overall diet quality.

Before the assessment of chronic salt exposure was made, the salt content of different salty snacks had been identified. A total of 48 different salty pre-packaged food products were analyzed and the selection of products represented 91% of all the products listed in the questionnaire. The salt content in selected snack products ranged from 0.9 g/100 g (nuts and seeds) to as much as 3.5 g/100 g in Clipsy® product. The analyzed values were in good correlation with the values specified on the product labels (r^2 = 0.924). The package weight ranged between 18 g and 200 g, depending on the type of salty snacks, and this parameter was of great importance for the potential salt intake in a student population (Table 4).

Table 4. Salt content in snack products.

Product Type and Description	Salt Content (g/100 g)	G (g)	Percentage of Participants Reporting Using Certain Type of Snack Products (%)
Bakery products (crackers, fish-shaped products, *bake rolls*® and *kubz*®, pretzels, sticks)	2.0–3.2 [a]/2.6 [b]	(18–160) [c]/44.6 [d]	31
Chips products (tortilla and potato)	1.3–1.6/1.5	(40–150)/46.9	20
Flips products (with peanuts, and classic)	1.4–2.4/1.9	(30–50)/23	7
Clipsy products®	1.7–3.5/2.6	45/45	7
Salted popcorn	1.5–1.9/1.7	(50–200)/90	20
Nuts and seeds	0.9–2.7/1.8	(42–200)/90	15

[a] range for salt content values; [b] average value of salt content; [c] range value of the package size (g); [d] average value of the package size (g).

Evaluation of dietary exposure to salt from various salty snack products consumed by the young population was conducted by analyzing a randomly selected sub-group of 200 participants during two slots of 72 h dietary recall (DR1 and DR2). The average exposure of students to salt from salty snack products was approximately 0.71 g/day (Figure 1). Maximum salt exposure from salty snack products was 2.8 g/day. Salt intake from snack products for the majority of participants ranged between 0.4 and 1 g/day, 33% of all participants were exposed to a daily salt intake below 0.5 g, whereas 18.5% of students showed exposure to salt above 1 g.

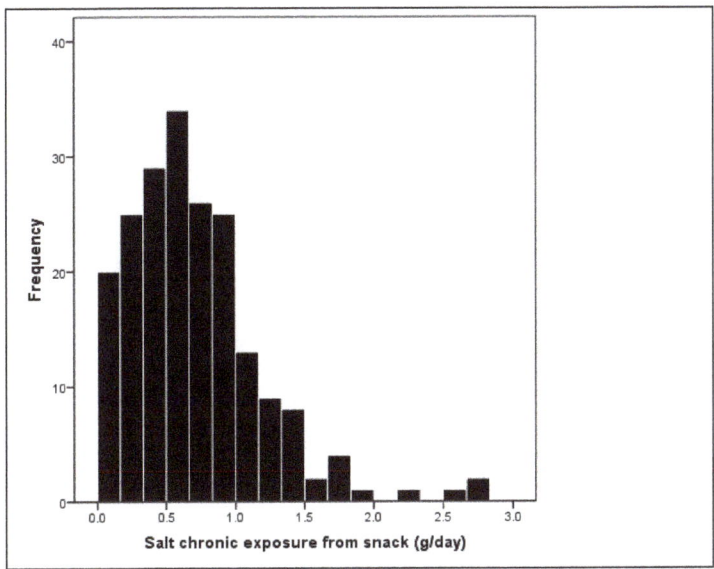

Figure 1. Salt chronic exposure from snack products regularly used among urban student population. N = number of participants.

4. Discussion

This study was the first to explore timing, frequency, and quantity of salty snack consumption and the factors associated with their usage among urban-living high-school and university students in this region and it indicated the notable potential of this food group for increasing daily salt intake. The products that were considered as salty snacks in this study were pre-packaged, available in markets, local shops or traffics near university/high-school, or from vending machines provided on school/university.

4.1. Questionnaire Reliability

Reliability analysis regarding internal consistency, so as inter-item correlation showed very good validity of the questionnaire used in this study. Multidimensionality of the questionnaire was analyzed by principal component analysis (PCA). PCA revealed several aspects of this questionnaire: pattern of salty snack consumption, influence of the label information on snack consumption, general dietary habits, and personal preferences which are related to salty snack usage. The four main layers of the questionnaire enabled analyzing snack usage habits of Serbian urban-living students and to make some general conclusions in order to improve eating habits. This also could open the additional exploration possibilities of presented results in PCA extracted factors as separate variables, and their relationship with different study data, but this direction would go beyond the basic aims of the current investigation and is certainly going to be exploited in the future.

4.2. General Characteristics of Salty Snack Consumption Patterns

In our study the consumption frequency in urban-living students generally varied from once per weak to several times per week. This is consistent with the results from the northern part of Serbia [17] and north Italy, where the mean weekly consumption of all snacks and salty snacks among students was several servings/week [18]. The findings of the 2016 statistical survey for Europe were similar with the frequency of eating salty snacks at least once a week in 75% of general population in Spain and United Kingdom, and 48% in Germany [19]. Home and evening as preferable location and time of day for salty snacking occasions were common for both student age groups. Similar preferences for Canadian young and adult population were found by Vatanparasat et al. [20]. Higher intake of these food items in the evening in both study groups could be attributed to their having more spare time, spending more time with friends at home or in front of the TV set/computer, or replacing dinner with these products.

Our results enabled testing if there was a correlation between salty snack consumption and the weight of participants. Despite the fact that in Serbia there is an upward trend in obesity among young people as revealed by the statistics of the Institute of Public Health, [21] our subjects from both study groups were of normal body composition (over 90%). Since the weight and height data were self-reported there is a possibility that some under-reporting was present. The "high snack intake group" had slightly lower BMI which could support the hypothesis that higher overall snacking frequency is not associated with the obesity risk in adolescents and young people. The results of other similar investigations of young people's eating behaviors vary [22–25]. Although Alphonso et al., found a positive correlation between the BMI and the snacking of chips, popcorn, salted peanuts, and crackers, [26] there was no correlation between the frequency of fast food, soft drink, and candy intake and BMI in the research conducted in the US, where those with a normal BMI consumed 1.1 salty snacks over a period of two days, while overweight, obese, and morbidly obese people consumed 0.9, 1.0, and 0.9 snacks [27]. The review paper of Williamson et al. also indicated that the available evidence do not support snacking as a significant factor leading to weight-related outcomes [28]. No definitive explanation for these findings has been offered, but the reason found in our study could be that the increased energy needs during the period of intensive growth and development were not fulfilled with regular diet, and that the energy contribution from salty snack food items does not exceed the recommended value for particular age. The hypothesis that the quality of overall nutrition may be insufficient to meet the energy needs of young people and consumption of savory snacks is one of the ways to achieve the required energy intake is supported by the fact that over 10% of the students covered by our study consumed salty snacks immediately after the main meal, which could mean that they did not feel satiation after eating. Other possible explanation is that high snack intake increases the feeling of satiety which may lead to skipping main meals and to the lower energy intake.

4.3. Factors Associated with High Frequency of Salty Snack Usage

The factors associated with the frequency of salty snack intake in the student urban-living population were investigated. More frequent snacking in all students was associated with day-periods intake, number of refreshments and self-perception towards diet quality ($p < 0.001$). The product type was also an important determinant for a more frequent consumption, which testifies to the relevance of taste factors among young population. Cross et al. [29] 25 years ago concluded that children and adolescents choose snack based on taste over nutrition and more often choose salty, crunchy foods. No correlation was found as regards the number of main meals and the motivation reasons, although some previous studies have found correlation between meal skipping and higher snacking frequency [1]. Additional determinants for increased salty snack frequency consumption in our study were younger age which indicates that younger students can be less prone to the health-conscious eating behavior. The correlation between snacking and gender in our study was not significant and mixed results are available from previous studies [1], although in some of them it was observed that women are often better informed about nutrition and are more inclined to making healthier food choices [30].

As far as the context of salty snacking is concerned, the students included in our study ate less salty snacks at school or faculty and rarely consumed snack food outdoors, which came as a surprise because some previous studies [31,32] revealed that many adolescents consume more snacks while in the company of their peers. The fact that the participants consumed salty snacks mostly at home is also significant for planning possible dietary interventions as it points to the importance of the parental role and the home food environment in replacing the existing dietary patterns with healthier ones. The home was also the most prevalent location for overall snacking in Canadian population [20].

4.4. Differences between High School and University Students

The investigated population of high-school students differed from that of university students in several aspects of snack consumption. A substantially higher number of high-school students were in the "high snack intake group" and also more likely to eat multiple packages of salty snacks. There were several reported comparisons between high-school and college participants related to snack usage and salty snack usage, with similar findings of decreasing consumption trend with student maturity [27]. This can be attributed to the greater maturity of university students, or the greater availability of canteens offering main meals at their faculties. A recent study has found that older students, especially in the university setting, are continuously prompted to make healthful food choices, which could also be the reason for a slightly healthier eating behavior [33].

When factors associated with high frequency of salty snack usage were analyzed separately for two student groups certain differences in influencing variables were noticed. Only in high-school student group significant predictor of high salty snack frequency intake was self-perception towards quality of their overall diet, so that better diet quality perception decreased chance for more frequent snack usage. We could assume that perceived poor diet quality in high-school students, at least in part was correlated to their more frequent salty snack use. The awareness of the nutritive value of salty snacks was more important variable for older students' high usage which was surprising because it was expected that paying attention to the nutritive information on the labels would lead to decreased snack consumption. One of the possible explanations for this finding could be that older students more frequently read the nutritive information but do not understand them properly and do not use them for making more informative food choices and this finding needs further investigation.

4.5. Contribution of Salty Snacks to Daily Salt Intake

In terms of potential contribution of salty snacks to the daily intake of salt, the average salt content in different snack types, the package size, and number of packages consumed were all important factors. The most frequently consumed salty snacks were those with the highest salt content (bakery products, flips, clipsy® products, and nuts/seeds). Likewise, taking into account that 40% of participating students consumed multiple snack packages on one snacking occasion, it could be assumed that students may intake significant amounts of salt from snacks. WHO recommends a daily salt intake of <5 g/day for individuals ≥16 years of age (recommended maximum level of intake, (RMLI)) [34]. According to several reports, the intake of salt among the Serbian population is far beyond the recommended amount, reaching 9 g/day and more [35,36] but the contribution of snacks was not previously evaluated. It was of interest to assess the average salt intake from salty snacks on a sample of Serbian urban-living students. The average calculated amount of salt intake from salty snack food represented 14.2% of RMLI, while 18.5% of participants had chronic salt intakes in excess of 20% RMLI only from this food group. If we acknowledge the aforementioned average salt intake for the Serbian population of 9 g/day, then salty snacks contributed an average of 7.9% to the total daily salt intake with a range of 0.22–31.1%. A systematic review of Menyanu et al. [37] identified bread, meat and meat products, sauces, spreads, and different fast foods as the major salt sources in the diets of low- and medium-income countries. Similar findings can be seen in the survey on the Members States' Implementation of the EU Salt Reduction Framework [38] with bread contributing to the total salt intake with ~20%, meat and meat products with 8–26%, and cheese and dairy products with 10%. If we make a comparison with the relevant data, it is evident that salty snack products could be an equally important food category in the diet of Serbian urban-living students as dairy products or even meat products and consequently they can significantly contribute to their overall salt intake. A recent study by Milincic et al. [39] revealed that 13.1% of adolescents in Serbia had moderately high blood pressure, 5.9% stage 1, and 3.5% stage 2 hypertension, whereas Milosevic Georgiev et al. [40] found elevated systolic blood pressure in 14.9% of Serbian students. Although the correlation between salt intake and hypertension in children and adolescents is still controversial, WHO recommends a reduction of salt intake to control blood pressure in this population [41]. This recommendation was confirmed by the European Salt Action Network in 2018 [42]. Our study indicates that snacking habits potentially represent easily modifiable health risk for urban student population and can be one of the targeted behaviors in adolescence to be dealt with in health management and salt reduction strategies.

4.6. Limitations and Implications

The strengths of this study include the range of young people from high school to university students and from different educational fields, and verification of FFQ data with a 72-h recall. The limitations of the study include possible variations in snack salt content, the magnitude of product category covered in the study, the self-reported height and weight, predominant female gender of participants, and a limited number of participants that completed two dietary recalls.

This research focused on snacking habits among young people in a developing country for which there is no sufficient data or applicable national policies and educational strategies. The study results demonstrated that salty snack products may be significant salt contributors for young people. The study important key points are that home environment and younger age population should be the focus of future educational and promotional strategies about healthier food choices. These findings are also useful for defining possible future product reformulation options.

5. Conclusions

In conclusion, the findings of this study provide the first information on dietary habits of urban-living students in Serbia connected to salty snacks consumption and their significant contribution to the salt daily intake. Identification of all important dietary sources of salt is in accordance with EU and WHO frameworks for salt reduction and the results of this study could present one important milestone in reduction salt initiatives on national level.

Supplementary Materials: The following are available online at http://www.mdpi.com/2072-6643/12/11/3290/s1, Table S1: Sample descriptive characteristics of study participants, Table S2: The rotated pattern matrix of the questionnaire scale. The four factors and their items, Table S3: Logistic regression analysis of the variables (questionnaire's items) that could predict a high level of salty snack product intake among the population of urban living students.

Author Contributions: All authors contributed to finalizing the manuscript. J.B.T. contributed to the study design, data collection, field work, interpretation of the data, and drafting of the manuscript. J.K.-S. contributed to data verification and statistical interpretation. H.B. contributed to checking the epidemiological methods and data presentations and discussion on epidemiological results. D.K. contributed to the verification of dietary methods, B.D. contributed to defining of study ethical issues and interpretation of data, and S.S. contributed to defining the goals, designing the study, and drafting the paper. All authors have read and agreed to the published version of the manuscript.

Funding: This study was financed by the grant from the Serbian Ministry of Education, Science and Technology Development (451-03-68/2020-14/200161).

Conflicts of Interest: The authors declare no conflict of interest. The funders had no role in the design of the study, collection, analyses, or interpretation of data, writing of the manuscript, or in the decision to publish the results.

Transparency Declaration: The lead author affirms that this manuscript is an honest, accurate, and transparent account of the study being reported. The lead author affirms that no important aspects of the study have been omitted and that any discrepancies from the study as planned have been explained.

Ethics Statement: The study was approved by the Ethics Committee for Biomedical Research of the Faculty of Pharmacy, University of Belgrade, Serbia, project identification code 164/3, and date of approval 25 February 2015.

References

1. Savige, G.; MacFarlane, A.; Ball, K.; Worsley, A.; Crawford, D. Snacking behaviours of adolescents and their association with skipping meals. *Int. J. Behav. Nutr. Phy.* **2007**, *4*, 36. [CrossRef]
2. Bellisle, F. Meals and snacking, diet quality and energy balance. *Physiol. Behav.* **2014**, *134*, 38–43. [CrossRef]
3. Piernas, C.; Popkin, B.M. Trends in snacking among US children. *Health Aff. Millwood* **2010**, *29*, 398–404. [CrossRef]
4. Ortiz-Hernandez, L.; Gomez-Tello, B.L. Food consumption in Mexican adolescents. *Rev. Panam. Salud Publica* **2008**, *24*, 127–135. [CrossRef]
5. National Institute for Public Health and the Environment; Ministry of Health, Welfare and Sport. *Food Consumption in The Netherlands and Its Determinants*; RIVM Report 2016-0195; National Institute for Public Health and the Environment: Amsterdam, The Netherlands, 2016; Available online: http://www.rivm.nl/bibliotheek/rapporten/2016-0195.pdf (accessed on 28 July 2020).
6. Llaurado, E.; Albar, S.A.; Giralt, M.; Evans, C.E.L. The effect of snacking and eating frequency on dietary quality in British adolescents. *Eur. J. Nutr.* **2016**, *55*, 1789. [CrossRef]
7. Palla, L.; Chapman, A.; Beh, E.; Pot, G.; Almiron-Roig, E. Where Do Adolescents Eat Less-Healthy Foods? Correspondence Analysis and Logistic Regression Results from the UK National Diet and Nutrition Survey. *Nutrients* **2020**, *12*, 2235. [CrossRef]
8. Van den Broek, N.; Larsen, J.K.; Verhagen, M.; Burk, W.J.; Vink, J.M. Is Adolescents' Food Intake Associated with Exposure to the Food Intake of Their Mothers and Best Friends? *Nutrients* **2020**, *12*, 786. [CrossRef]
9. Pries, A.M.; Huffman, S.L.; Champeny, M.; Adhikary, I.; Benjamin, M.; Coly, A.N.; Diop, E.H.I.; Mengkheang, K.; Sy, N.Y.; Dhungel, S.; et al. Consumption of commercially produced snack foods and sugar sweetened beverages during the complementary feeding period in four African and Asian urban contexts. *Matern. Child. Nutr.* **2017**, *13*, e12412. [CrossRef] [PubMed]
10. Samuelson, G. Dietary habits and nutritional status in adolescents over Europe. An overview of current studies in the Nordic countries. *Eur. J. Clin. Nutr.* **2000**, *54* (Suppl. 1), S21–S28. [CrossRef]
11. Gordon, B.R. *Snack Food*, 1st ed.; Springer: New York, NY, USA, 1990; pp. 25–284. ISBN 978-1-4613-1477-6.
12. Ponzo, V.; Ganzit, G.P.; Soldati, L.; de Carli, I.; Fanzola, I.; Maiandi, M.; Durazzo, M.; Bo, S. Blood pressure and sodium intake from snacks in adolescents. *Eur. J. Clin. Nutr.* **2015**, *69*, 681–686. [CrossRef]
13. World Health Organization (WHO). Shake the Salt Habit. 2016. Available online: https://www.who.int/dietphysicalactivity/publications/shake-salt-habit/en/ (accessed on 23 September 2020).

14. WHO. *BMI Classification*; WHO: Geneva, Switzerland, 2017. Available online: https://www.euro.who.int/en/health-topics/disease-prevention/nutrition/a-healthy-lifestyle/body-mass-index-bmi (accessed on 24 July 2020).
15. Hortiz, W. *Official Methods of Analysis of AOAC International*, 17th ed.; AOAC International: Rockville, MD, USA, 2000.
16. National Institute for Public Health and the Environment; Ministry of Health, Welfare and Sport. *Probabilistic Dietary Exposure Models*; RIVM Letter report 2015-0191; National Institute for Public Health and the Environment: Amsterdam, The Netherlands, 2015. Available online: https://www.rivm.nl/bibliotheek/rapporten/2015-0191.pdf (accessed on 29 July 2020).
17. Požar, H.; Požar, Č. Adolescent Eating Behavior in the Secondary Medical School in Novi Sad and the Technical School in Subotica. *Hrana I Ishr.* **2017**, *58*, 30–37. [CrossRef]
18. Lupi, S.; Bagordo, F.; Stefanati, A.; Grassi, T.; Piccinni, L.; Bergamini, M.; de Donno, A. Assessment of lifestyle and eating habits among undergraduate students in northern Italy. *Ann. Ist. Super. Sanità* **2015**, *51*, 154–161. [CrossRef] [PubMed]
19. Statista. The Statistics Portal. In *Frequency of Eating Salty Snacks at Least Once per Week in Selected Countries in the European Union (EU) in 2016*; Statista 2020: Hamburg, Germany, 2020. Available online: https://www.statista.com/statistics/627178/frequency-of-eating-salty-snacks-european-union-eu/ (accessed on 4 August 2020).
20. Vatanparasat, H.; Islam, N.; Masoodi, H.; Shafiee, M.; Patil, R.P.; Smith, J.; Whiting, S.J. Time, location and frequency of snack consumption in different agr groups of Canadians. *Nutr. J.* **2020**, *19*, 85. [CrossRef]
21. Institute of Public Health of Serbia "Dr Milan Jovanović Batut". *Health of Population of Serbia, Analytical Study 1997–2007*; Institute of Public Health of Serbia "Dr Milan Jovanović Batut": Beograd, Serbia, 2009. Available online: http://www.batut.org.rs/download/publikacije/Health%20of%20population%201997-2007.pdf (accessed on 2 August 2020).
22. Alkhamis, A. *The Relationship between Snacking Patterns and Body Mass Index in College Students*; University of Wisconsin-Stout: Menomonie, WI, USA, 2011. Available online: https://pdfs.semanticscholar.org/339e/9e5e90a78c77215bbba1f2b414191745609c.pdf (accessed on 28 July 2020).
23. Tanton, J.; Dodd, L.J.; Woodfield, L.; Mabhala, M. Eating Behaviours of British University Students: A Cluster Analysis on a Neglected Issue. *Adv. Prev. Med.* **2015**, *2015*, 639239. [CrossRef]
24. Al-Hazzaa, H.M.; Abahussain, N.A.; Al-Sobayel, H.I.; Qahwaji, D.M.; Alsulaiman, N.A.; Musaiger, A.O. Prevalence of Overweight, Obesity, and Abdominal Obesity among Urban Saudi Adolescents: Gender and Regional Variations. *J. Health Popul. Nutr.* **2014**, *32*, 634–645.
25. Niven, P.; Scully, M.; Morley, B.; Baur, L.; Crawford, D.; Pratt, I.A.; Wakefield, M. What factors are associated with frequent unhealthy snack-food consumption among Australian secondary-school students? *Pub. Health Nutr.* **2014**, *18*, 2153–2160. [CrossRef]
26. Alphonso, G. *Nutritional Knowledge, Attitude, Behaviors and Anthropometric Data Among Adolescent Female Secondary School Students*; University of West Indies (Jamaica): A Research Paper; ID 810000372; University of West Indies (Jamaica): Kingston, Jamaica, 2013. Available online: https://uwispace.sta.uwi.edu/dspace/bitstream/handle/2139/41726/Alphonso_G_UWIAgriExt_Undergrad_ResearchProj.pdf?sequence=1&isAllowed=y (accessed on 2 August 2020).
27. Just, D.R.; Wansink, B. Fast food, soft drink and candy intake is unrelated to body mass index for 95% of American adults. *Obes. Sci. Pract.* **2015**, *1*, 126–130. [CrossRef]
28. Williamson, V.G.; Dilip, A.; Dillard, J.R.; Morgan-Daniel, J.; Lee, A.M.; Cardel, M.I. The Influence of Socioeconomic Status on Snacking and Weight among Adolescents: A Scoping Review. *Nutrients* **2020**, *12*, 167. [CrossRef]
29. Cross, A.T.; Babicz, D.; Cushman, D. Snacking patterns among 1,800 adults and children. *J. Am. Diet. Assoc.* **1994**, *94*, 1398–1403. [CrossRef]
30. Arganini, C.; Saba, A.; Comitato, R.; Virgili, F.; Turrini, A. Gender Differences in Food Choice and Dietary Intake in Modern Western Societies. In *Public Health—Social and Behavioral Health*; Intech Open: London, UK, 2012. Available online: http://cdn.intechopen.com/pdfs/36935/InTech-Gender_differences_in_food_choice_and_dietary_intake_in_modern_western_societies.pdf (accessed on 15 July 2020).
31. Wouters, E.J.; Larsen, J.K.; Kremers, S.P.; Dagnelie, P.C.; Geenen, R. Peer influence on snacking behavior in adolescence. *Appetite* **2010**, *55*, 11–17. [CrossRef]

32. Story, M.; Sztainer, D.N.; French, S. Individual and Environmental Influences on Adolescent Eating Behaviors. *J. Am. Diet Assoc.* **2002**, *102*, 40–51. [CrossRef]
33. Deliens, T.; Clarys, P.; de Bourdeaudhuij, I.; Deforche, B. Determinants of eating behaviour in university students: A qualitative study using focus group discussions. *BMC Public Health* **2014**, *14*, 53–65. [CrossRef] [PubMed]
34. WHO. Sodium Intake for Adults and Children. 2014. Available online: https://www.who.int/nutrition/publications/guidelines/sodium_intake_printversion.pdf (accessed on 18 June 2020).
35. Powles, J.; Fahimi, S.; Micha, R.; Khatibzadeh, S.; Shi, P.; Ezzati, M.; Engell, R.E.; Lim, S.S.; Danaei, G.; Mozaffarian, D. BMJ Global, regional and national sodium intakes in 1990 and 2010: A systematic analysis of 24 h urinary sodium excretion and dietary surveys worldwide. *BMJ Open* **2013**, *3*, e003733. [CrossRef] [PubMed]
36. Jovičić, J.; Grujičić, M.; Rađen, S.; Novaković, B. Sodium intake and dietary sources of sodium in a sample of undergraduate students from Novi Sad, Serbia. *Vojnosanit. Pregl.* **2016**, *73*, 651–656. [CrossRef]
37. Menyanu, E.; Russell, J.; Charlton, K. Dietary Sources of Salt in Low- and Middle-Income Countries: A Systematic Literature Review. *Int. J. Environ. Res. Public Health* **2019**, *16*, 2082. [CrossRef]
38. Survey on the Members States' Implementation of the EU Salt Reduction Framework. 2012. Available online: https://ec.europa.eu/health/sites/health/files/nutrition_physical_activity/docs/salt_report1_en.pdf (accessed on 16 August 2020).
39. Milincic, Z.; Nikolic, D.; Simeunovic, S.; Novakovic, I.; Petronic, I.; Risimic, D.; Simeunovic, D. School children systolic and diastolic blood pressure values: YUSAD study. *Cent. Eur. J. Med.* **2011**, *6*, 634–639. [CrossRef]
40. Milosevic-Georgiev, A.; Krajnovic, D.; Kotur-Stevuljevic, J.; Ignjatovic, S.; Marinkovic, V. Undiagnosed hyperglycemia and hypertension as indicators of the vascular risk factors of future cardiovascular disease among population of Serbian students. *J. Med. Biochem.* **2018**, *37*, 289–298. [CrossRef]
41. WHO. *Reducing Sodium Intake to Control Blood Pressure in Children*; WHO: Geneva, Switzerland, 2019; Available online: https://www.who.int/elena/titles/sodium_bp_children/en/ (accessed on 8 August 2020).
42. WHO, Regional office for Europe. *European Salt Action Network Restates Its Support for WHO Goal of Reducing Salt Intake to 5 g per Day or Less*; WHO: Geneva, Switzerland, 2018. Available online: http://www.euro.who.int/en/health-topics/disease-prevention/nutrition/news/news/2018/12/european-salt-action-network-restates-its-support-for-who-goal-of-reducing-salt-intake-to-5-g-per-day-or-less (accessed on 19 August 2020).

Publisher's Note: MDPI stays neutral with regard to jurisdictional claims in published maps and institutional affiliations.

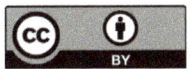

© 2020 by the authors. Licensee MDPI, Basel, Switzerland. This article is an open access article distributed under the terms and conditions of the Creative Commons Attribution (CC BY) license (http://creativecommons.org/licenses/by/4.0/).

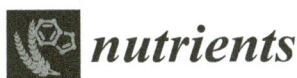

Article

Nutritional Status and Oral Frailty: A Community Based Study

Yoshiaki Nomura [1,*], Yoshimasa Ishii [2], Shunsuke Suzuki [2], Kenji Morita [2], Akira Suzuki [2], Senichi Suzuki [2], Joji Tanabe [2], Yasuo Ishiwata [2], Koji Yamakawa [2], Yota Chiba [2], Meu Ishikawa [1], Kaoru Sogabe [1], Erika Kakuta [3], Ayako Okada [4], Ryoko Otsuka [1] and Nobuhiro Hanada [1]

1. Department of Translational Research, Tsurumi University School of Dental Medicine, Yokohama 230-8501, Japan; ishikawa-me@tsurumi-u.ac.jp (M.I.); sogabe-k@tsurumi-u.ac.jp (K.S.); otsuka-ryoko@tsurumi-u.ac.jp (R.O.); hanada-n@tsurumi-u.ac.jp (N.H.)
2. Ebina Dental Association, Kanagawa 243-0421, Japan; ishiiryo141@gmail.com (Y.I.); shun-s@wg8.so-net.ne.jp (S.S.); morita-d-c-2@t06.itscom.net (K.M.); suzuki@bell-dental.com (A.S.); lion@kd5.so-net.ne.jp (S.S.); tanabedental5@me.com (J.T.); yasuo-i@rb3.so-net.ne.jp (Y.I.); cherry@cherry-dental.com (K.Y.); yota@db3.so-net.ne.jp (Y.C.)
3. Department of Oral Microbiology, Tsurumi University School of Dental Medicine, Yokohama 230-8501, Japan; kakuta-erika@tsurumi-u.ac.jp
4. Department of Operative Dentistry, Tsurumi University School of Dental Medicine, Yokohama 230-8501, Japan; okada-a@tsurumi-u.ac.jp
* Correspondence: nomura-y@tsurumi-u.ac.jp

Received: 19 August 2020; Accepted: 17 September 2020; Published: 21 September 2020

Abstract: Compromised oral health can alter food choices. Poor masticatory function leads to imbalanced food intake and undesirable nutritional status. The associations among nutritional status, oral health behavior, and self-assessed oral functions status were investigated using a community-based survey. In total, 701 subjects more than 50 years old living Ebina city located southwest of the capital Tokyo were investigated. The number of remaining teeth was counted by dental hygienists. Oral health behavior and self-assessed oral functions were evaluated by oral frailty checklist. Nutritional status was evaluated by the brief-type self-administered diet history questionnaire using Dietary Reference Intakes for Japanese as reference. More than 80% of subjects' intakes of vitamin B_{12}, pantothenic acid, copper, and proteins were sufficient. In contrast, only 19% of subjects' intake of vitamin A was sufficient and 35.5% for vitamin B_1. More than 90% of subjects' intakes of vitamin D and vitamin K were sufficient. Only 35.5% of subjects' intakes of dietary fiber were sufficient. Overall, 88.9% of subjects had excess salt. The number of remaining teeth was not correlated with nutritional intakes. Oral health behavior significantly correlated with nutritional intakes. Oral functions are important for food choice; however, oral functions were not directly correlated with nutritional intakes. Comprehensive health instructions including nutrition and oral health education is necessary for health promotion.

Keywords: nutritional status; population survey; oral frailty; health behavior

1. Introduction

Compromised oral health status can alter food choices, leading to suboptimal nutritional status. The associations among dietary practices, nutritional status, and oral health status are complex with many interrelated factors.

Oral health status is associated with various diseases and quality of life. Two main pathways have been suggested for the relationship between oral health status and general health: odontogenic bacteremia [1,2] and malnutrition by deteriorated masticatory function [3–5]. Mastication is an important function of the oral cavity. Masticatory function is strongly suggested to be associated with general health. Decreased masticatory function changes food preferences and disturbs balance of food intake [6,7]. In older persons, the number of teeth affects the intake of some foods and nutrients [8,9]. Poor masticatory function leads to imbalanced food intake and undesirable nutritional status that can lead to chronic systemic illness. Especially in older persons, a relationship between masticatory function and mortality has been suggested [10,11].

Oral frailty is defined as a mild decline in oral function, and it is reversible in the early stage. Therefore, early detection and treatment of oral frailty is very useful. Prevention of oral frailty can be expected to reduce medical and nursing care cost. Fewer than 20 remaining teeth, articulatory oral motor skill, weak tongue pressure, difficulties eating tough foods, and difficulties in swallowing tea or soup are risk factors for physical frailty, sarcopenia, and disability [12]. Therefore, the concept of oral frailty was widely introduced in Japan [12,13].

Fermentable carbohydrate, especially sugar, causes dental caries, and thus the relationship between sugar intake and dental caries has been intensively studied. Dental researchers were involved as guideline editors for sugar intake published by World Health Organization [14]. However, studies on the relationship among oral health status, nutritional status, and nutrient intake other than sugar consumption are still insufficient [15,16]. Poor dietary intake increased the risk of periodontal disease. Inverse associations were found between fatty acids, vitamin C, vitamin E, beta-carotene, fiber, calcium, dairy, fruits, and vegetables and risk of periodontal disease [17]. The relationship between oral health and nutrition is primarily related to masticatory function, but it is complicated by other factors such as race, culture, lifestyle, and personal preferences [18,19].

The basic health policy of the Japanese government is to prevent the onset and aggravation of major noncommunicable diseases as well as frailty in older persons. Insufficient or imbalanced nutritional intake is one of the major common risk factors for the noncommunicable diseases and frailty. "Dietary Reference Intakes for Japanese" was formulated and has been revised every five years under the Health Promotion Act [20,21]. Target values have been set for the purpose of maintaining/promoting health, preventing the onset and progression of noncommunicable diseases, and prevention of malnutrition and frailty in the elderly. The target values for each of the nutrients are set according to the gender and age groups. Meeting these values is desirable to prevent non-communicable diseases and frailty.

For the assessment of nutritional intake for Japanese people, a validated questionnaire has been developed and named as the brief-type self-administered diet history questionnaire (BDHQ) [22–25]. BDHQ has been generally used in epidemiological studies carried out in Japan from elementary school children to older Japanese [22–25].

Few studies have investigated the relationship between oral functions and nutritional status [26]. In this study, the number of remaining teeth was recorded, while self-assessed oral functions and nutritional intake on a community basis were investigated using BDHQ and evaluated using the Dietary Reference Intakes for Japanese, respectively. The purpose of this study was to examine the impact of oral frailty on nutrient intake levels and nutrient intake at a community level.

2. Materials and Methods

2.1. Setting

A questionnaire on oral frail was distributed for the citizens of Ebina city, located near the capital of Tokyo. A booth was set for the survey outside of city hall, a housing estate, and a sports center from December 2018 to January 2019. Before distribution, age was asked. The questionnaire was distributed to subjects more than 50 years old. In the booth, dental hygienists counted the number of remaining teeth under the supervision of dentists. We recommended all subjects visit a dental office. Fifty-five subjects (7.8%) agreeing to visit a dental office were invited to a dental office and the number of remaining teeth were again counted. The representativeness of the participants in this study was confirmed by comparing three major nutrient intakes and self-reported number of remaining teeth obtained from the Japanese national health and nutrition examination survey conducted at 2018 [27].

2.2. Questionnaire

The oral frailty checklist proposed by the Japan dental association was used. The checklist consisted by 8 items: (1) harder to eat hard food than half a year ago (difficult to eat hard food); (2) sometimes choke on tea or soup (choking); (3) do you use dentures (using denture); (4) minding about oral dryness (Xerostomia); (5) less frequently going out than half a year ago (less frequently going out); (6) capable of chewing hard food such as pickled radish or shredded and dried squid (feasible to chew hard food); (7) brushing teeth at least twice a day (brushing teeth at least twice a day); and (8) attending dentist at least once a year (regular attendance of dental clinic).

By the standard protocol, if subjects answered yes to Item 1, 2 or 3, two points were given for each answer. If subjects answered yes to Item 4, 5 or 6, one point was given for each answer. If subjects answered no to Item 7, 8 or 9, one point was given for each answer. The maximum score was 11. The screening criterion was defined by the sum of the scores: Low risk for 0–2 points, moderate risk for 3 points, and high risk for more than 4 points.

2.3. Dietary Reference Intakes for Japanese (2015)

Japanese Minister of Health, Labor and Welfare formulated Dietary Reference Intakes for Japanese are in accordance with Article 30-2 of the Health Promotion Act (Act No. 103 of 2002) [20,21]. It proposes target values of desirable dietary intake of energy and nutrients for Japanese people to maintain and promote their health. Dietary reference intakes (DRIs) were determined based on scientific findings where data were available. It determined reference values for 34 nutrients and energy intakes.

For nutrients, five reference values were determined: Estimated Average Requirement (EAR), Recommended Dietary Allowance (RDA), Adequate Intake (AI), Tolerable Upper Intake Level (UL), and Tentative Dietary Goal for preventing LRDs (DG).

The EARs indicate the amount that would meet the nutrient requirements of 50% of the population. The RDA indicates the amount that would meet the requirement of most of the population. The Adequate Intake (AI) was developed where EAR and RDA could not be set due to insufficient scientific evidence. For the purpose of avoiding adverse health effects due to excessive intake, Tolerable Upper Intake Level (UL) was determined. For the purpose of prevention of Lifestyle-Related Diseases (LRDs), Tentative Dietary Goal for preventing LRDs (DG) was developed. Reference values were determined separately with respect to gender and age group.

Target BMI range is presented in this Dietary Reference Intakes for Japanese. Target BMI range is presented by age groups, and it is common to men and women: 20.0–24.9 (kg/m^2) for 50–69 years old, 21.5–24.9 (kg/m^2) for 70 years older.

2.4. Brief-Type Self-Administered Diet History Questionnaire (BDHQ)

For the evaluation of the nutritional status, the brief-type self-administered diet history questionnaire (BDHQ) was used. The BDHQ asks about the consumption frequency of selected foods to estimate the dietary intake of fifty-eight food and beverage items during the preceding month. Details of the BDHQ's structure, method of calculating dietary intake are described by its developers [16–20]. Calculation of nutritional intakes was ordered from the DHQ support center (Gender Medical Research, Co. Ltd., Tokyo, Japan).

Calculated nutritional status was classified by the target values by Dietary Reference Intakes for Japanese [20,21].

2.5. Examinations

In the survey booth, the number of remaining teeth was counted by a dental hygienist using penlight, disposable dental mirror, and probe. Height and body weight were measured. Body Mass Index (BMI) was calculated by the following formula:

$$BMI = body\ weight\ (kg) \div (body\ height\ (m))^2 \tag{1}$$

2.6. Statistical Analysis

Descriptive analysis was performed by SPSS version 24.0 (IBM, Tokyo, Japan). For contentious variables, normality was checked by Kolmogorov–Smirnov test. For the comparisons of groups, t-test, Mann–Whitney U test, or Kruskal–Wallis test was applied by the normality of distribution. To visualize correlations, structural equation modeling (SEM) was carried out by AMOS version 24.0 (IBM, Tokyo, Japan).

2.7. Ethics

Informed written consent was obtained simultaneously at the time of collection of questionnaire. The study protocol was approved by the Ethical Committee of Tsurumi University School of Dental Medicine (approval number: 1747).

3. Results

3.1. Characteristics of the Participants

The distribution and collection of the questionnaire was conducted simultaneously. Therefore, all questionnaires were collected. The data of 701 subjects (351 men, 350 women, mean age 71.5 ± 8.9) were analyzed. Their numbers and proportion in age groups were: 50–59 years old, 49 (7.0%) for men and 40 (5.7%) for women; 60–69 years old, 99 (14.1%) for men and 97 (13.8%) for women; 70–79 years old, 148 (21.1%) for men and 149 (21.3%) for women; and more than 80 years old, 55 (7.8%) for men and 64 (9.1%) for women.

The results of the representativeness comparing Japanese national health and nutritional survey are shown in Table S1.

3.2. Nutritional Status and Body Mass Index

3.2.1. Proportion of Energy Intake and Body Mass Index (BMI)

Energy balance on three major nutrients are set in Dietary Reference Intakes for Japanese as Tentative Dietary Goal for preventing lifestyle related diseases (DG). Subjects within DG range were 70.5% for proteins, 54.9% for fats, and 36.8% for carbohydrates. The results are shown in Figure 1. When comparing men and women, the distributions were all statistically significant (BMI, proteins, and fats, $p < 0.01$; carbohydrates, $p = 0.014$).

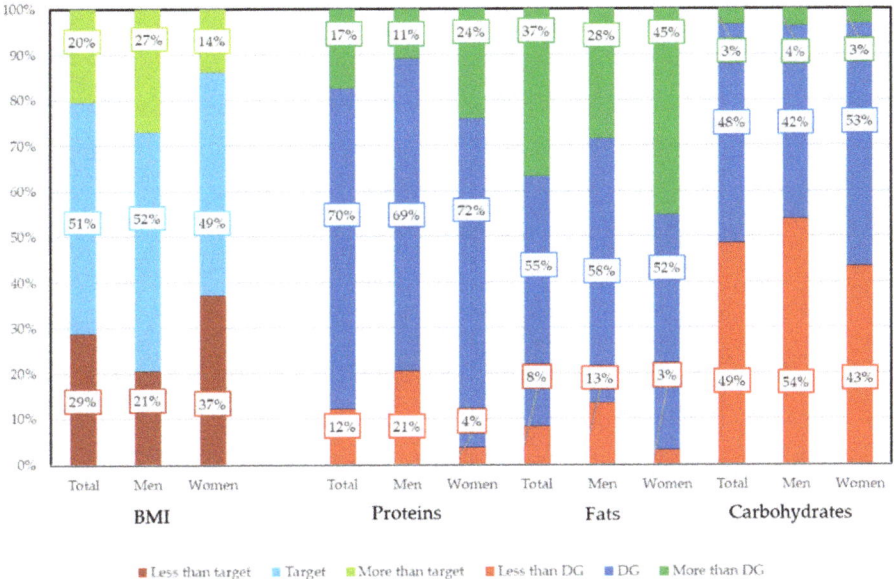

Figure 1. Proportion of subjects for BMI and meeting Tentative Dietary Goal for preventing lifestyle related diseases. Energy balance on three major nutrients are set in Dietary Reference Intakes for Japanese as Tentative Dietary Goal for preventing lifestyle related diseases (DG). DG for three major nutrients are expressed by percent of energy intakes. When comparing men and women, distributions were all statistically significant by χ^2 tests. Target BMI ranges are 20.0–24.9 (kg/m^2) for 50–69 years old and 21.5–24.9 (kg/m^2) for 70 years or older. Target BMI range is common to men and women. Optimal range of Body Mass Index (Target BMI) and Tentative Dietary Goal for preventing lifestyle related diseases (DG) are set in Dietary Reference Intakes for Japanese.

The three major nutrients (proteins, fats, and carbohydrates) of DG are set as energy balance by the ratio of energy intake. For proteins, 75% of subjects were in the DG range (13–20%); 36.6% of subjects exceeded the DG range (20–30%) of fats; and 48.6% were less than the DG range (50–65%) for carbohydrates. The proportion of woman with less than target value of BMI was higher than men. Proportion of men with more than target value of BMI was higher than women. The proportion of men whose intakes of macronutrients were less than TG was higher than women. The proportion of women whose intakes of proteins and fats were more than TG was higher than women.

There were 356 subjects within target BMI (50.8%). Scatter plots of BMI against the proportion of energy intakes are shown in Figure S2. Negative correlations were observed for three nutrients against BMI, and the statistically significant correlations were observed between proteins and BMI and between carbohydrate and BMI. However, the correlations were very weak: protein = −0.096 ($p = 0.011$), fats = −0.041($p = 0.283$), and carbohydrates = −0.138 ($p < 0.001$).

Cross tabulation of BMI and three macronutrients by categorize values by DG and target value is shown in Table 1. p-values except for Fats were statistically significant (proteins, $p = 0.017$; fats, $p = 0.091$; carbohydrates, $p = 0.002$). For continuous variables, p-values except for Fats were statistically significant. Differences in the number of remaining teeth, BMI, and the three macronutrients by categorical values of DG are shown in Table S2.

Table 1. BMI and three macronutrients intakes.

Nutrients	Cut Off	n	<Target	Target Range	Target<	p-Value	Mean SD	Median 25th–75th	p-Value
Proteins (%)	<DG	85	20	37	28		23.5 ± 3.4 *	23.4 (20.8–25.7)	
	DG	494	147	249	98	0.017	22.7 ± 3.1	22.5 (20.5–24.5)	0.032
	DG<	122	35	70	17		24.2 ± 22.4 *	23.2 (20.8–23.6)	
Fats (%)	<DG	58	14	24	20		23.5 ± 3.3	23.7 (20.5–25.6)	
	DG	385	113	196	76	0.091	22.6 ± 3.1	22.6 (20.6–24.5)	0.062
	DG<	258	75	136	47		22.6 ± 3.2	22.4 (20.6–24.1)	
Carbohydrates (%)	<DG	341	75	187	79		23.1 ± 3.1 **	22.9 (21.1–24.7)	
	DG	336	116	160	60	0.002	22.3 ± 3.2 **	22.2 (20.3–24.1)	0.003
	DG<	24	11	9	4		22.2 ± 3.2	21.7 (20.1–24.0)	

p values were calculated by χ^2 tests and Kruskal–Wallis tests. Target BMI ranges are 20.0–24.9 (kg/m^2) for 50–69 years old and 21.5–24.9 (kg/m^2) for 70 years or older. Target BMI range is common to men and women. * and ** statistically significant difference by multiple comparison of Dann–Bonferroni method, * $p = 0.036$, ** $p = 0.002$. DG—Tentative Dietary Goal for preventing lifestyle related diseases.

3.2.2. Vitamins, Macro Minerals, and Micro Minerals

The intakes of vitamins, macro minerals, and micro minerals were categorized by EAR (Estimated Average Requirement) and RDA (Recommended Dietary Allowance) or AI (Adequate Intake) according to Dietary Reference Intakes for Japanese (2015). Figure 2 shows the proportion of subjects whose intake of each nutrient was sufficient based on EAR and RDA (Figure 2A) and AI (Figure 2B). Additionally, fiber, which only has a DG set, is also presented. More than 80% of subjects' intakes of vitamin B_{12}, pantothenic acid, copper, and proteins were sufficient. In contrast, only 19% of subjects' intakes of vitamin A and 35.5% of subjects' intakes of vitamin B_1 were sufficient. More than 90% of subjects' intakes of vitamin D and vitamin K were sufficient. Only 35.5% of subjects' intakes of dietary fiber were sufficient. Sodium is converted as kitchen salts and a DG set. Overall, 88.9% of subjects had excess salt.

3.3. Oral Health Status of the Participants

The number of remaining teeth of the subjects participated in this study was 20.8 ±8.4 for men (median, 24; 25th–75th, 17–27), 21.6 ± 7.6 for women, (median, 24; 25th–75th, 19–27), and 21.22 ± 8.02 for total (median, 24; 25th–75th, 18–27). The difference was not statistically significant by Mann–Whitney U test. The proportion of subjects with more than 20 remaining teeth was 70.0% for men, 73.9% for women, and 72.0% for total.

The results of oral frailty screening questionnaire are summarized in Table 2.

Table 2. Frequency of the items of oral frailly scorning questionnaire.

Item of Oral Frailly Scorning Questionnaire	No N	No %	Yes N	Yes %	Missing N	Missing %
Difficult to eat hard food	572	81.6	127	18.1	2	0.3
Choking	595	84.9	102	14.6	4	0.6
Using denture	371	52.9	323	46.1	7	1.0
Xerostomia	528	75.3	171	24.4	2	0.3
Less frequently going out	571	81.5	127	18.1	3	0.4
Feasible to chew hard food	603	86.0	96	13.7	2	0.3
Brushing teeth at least twice a day	542	77.3	157	22.4	2	0.3
Regular attendance of dental clinic	513	73.2	183	26.1	5	0.7

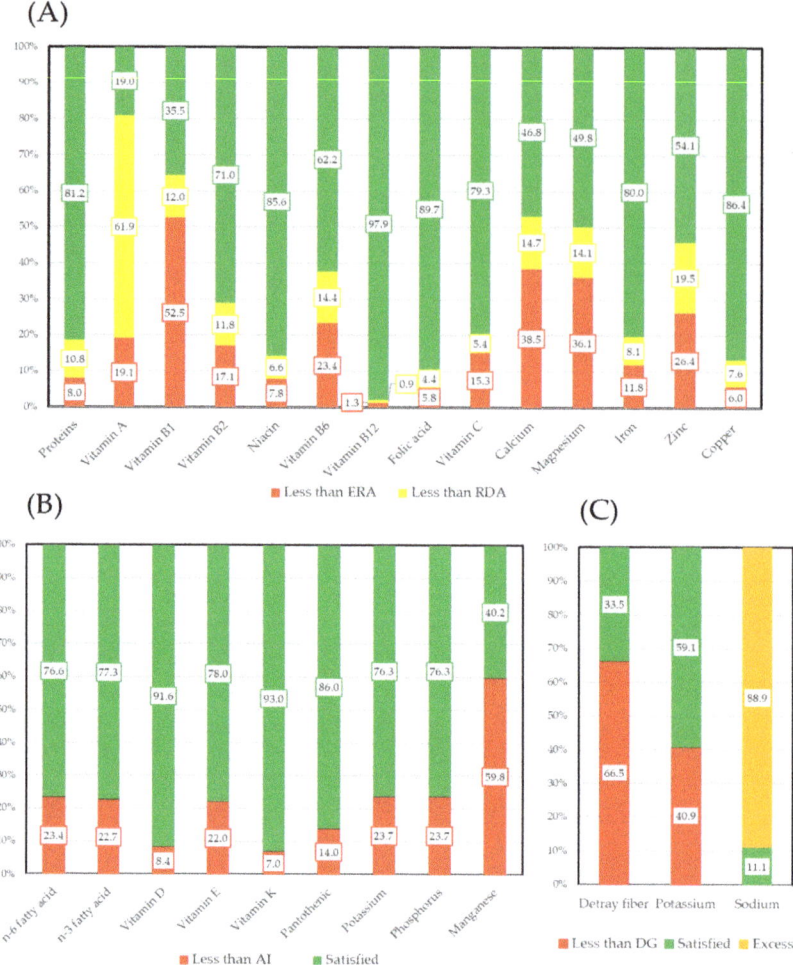

Figure 2. Meeting of vitamins, macro minerals, and micro minerals. Levels were determined by Dietary Reference Intakes for Japanese. Figure 2 shows the proportion of subjects whose intake of each nutrient was sufficient based (**A**) EAR and RDA. (**B**) AI. (**C**) DG. EAR: Estimated Average Requiremen. RDA: Recommended Dietary Allowance. AI: Adequate Intake. DG: Tentative Dietary Goal for preventing LRDs.

3.4. Oral Health Status and Nutritional Status

Oral frailty screening questionnaire consisted of eight items. The cross tabulations of response of these items and satisfied level nutrients are shown in Table S3. Additionally, the statistical significance of the net value of intakes of nutrients are shown in Table S4. As shown Table S3, oral frailty risk by screening of oral health questionnaire was statistically significant for 10 nutrients by χ^2 tests. For each item of the questionnaire, brushing teeth twice a day had significant correlations with 20 nutrients and having family dentist had significant correlation with 23 nutrients. In contrast, other items of the questionnaire had correlation with no or only one nutrient (Table S4). A similar tendency could be observed when using the net value of the intakes of nutrients, as shown in Table S4. The number of remaining teeth was only statistically significant for fiber. The results of Structured Equation Modeling

(SEM) are shown in Figure 3. All paths were statistically significant except for the path oral behavior to brushing teeth twice a day in the three major nutrients. Paths from oral behavior to nutrients intakes and oral behavior to brushing teeth twice a day and having regular dentist had similar values for water-soluble vitamins, fat-soluble vitamins, macro minerals, and micro minerals. In the model for three major nutrients, the path form oral health behavior to nutrients intakes were smaller than those in other nutrients. The effects of oral behavior on nutrition intakes were different between three major nutrients and other nutrients.

All paths were statistically significant except for the path oral behavior to brushing teeth twice a day in (Figure 3a). Paths from oral behavior to nutrients intakes and oral behavior to brushing teeth twice a day and having regular dentist have similar values in Figure 3b–e. In the model for three macronutrients, the path form oral health behavior to nutrients intakes was smaller than those in Figure 3b–e. The effects of oral behavior to nutrition intakes were different between three macronutrients and other nutrients.

Additionally, the energy balance of three macronutrients regulated by DG were analyzed. The results of cross tabulation by oral health behavior and energy balance of three major nutrients are shown in Table 3. By chi-square tests, energy balance of proteins and fats had a statistically significant correlation with brushing teeth twice a day. However, having a family dentist had no correlation with the energy balance of the three macronutrients.

Table 3. Oral health behavior and three macronutrients meets.

		Brushing Teeth at Least Twice a Day			Regular Attendance of Dental Clinic		
		No	Yes	p-Value	No	Yes	p-Value
Proteins	<DG	31	54	0.001	25	60	0.778
	DG	109	383		127	362	
	DG<	17	105		31	91	
Fats	<DG	21	36	0.006	21	36	0.153
	DG	90	294		99	282	
	DG<	46	212		63	195	
Carbohydrates	<DG	74	267	0.419	86	254	0.085
	DG	75	259		86	246	
	DG<	8	16		11	13	

p-values were calculated by Chi-square tests.

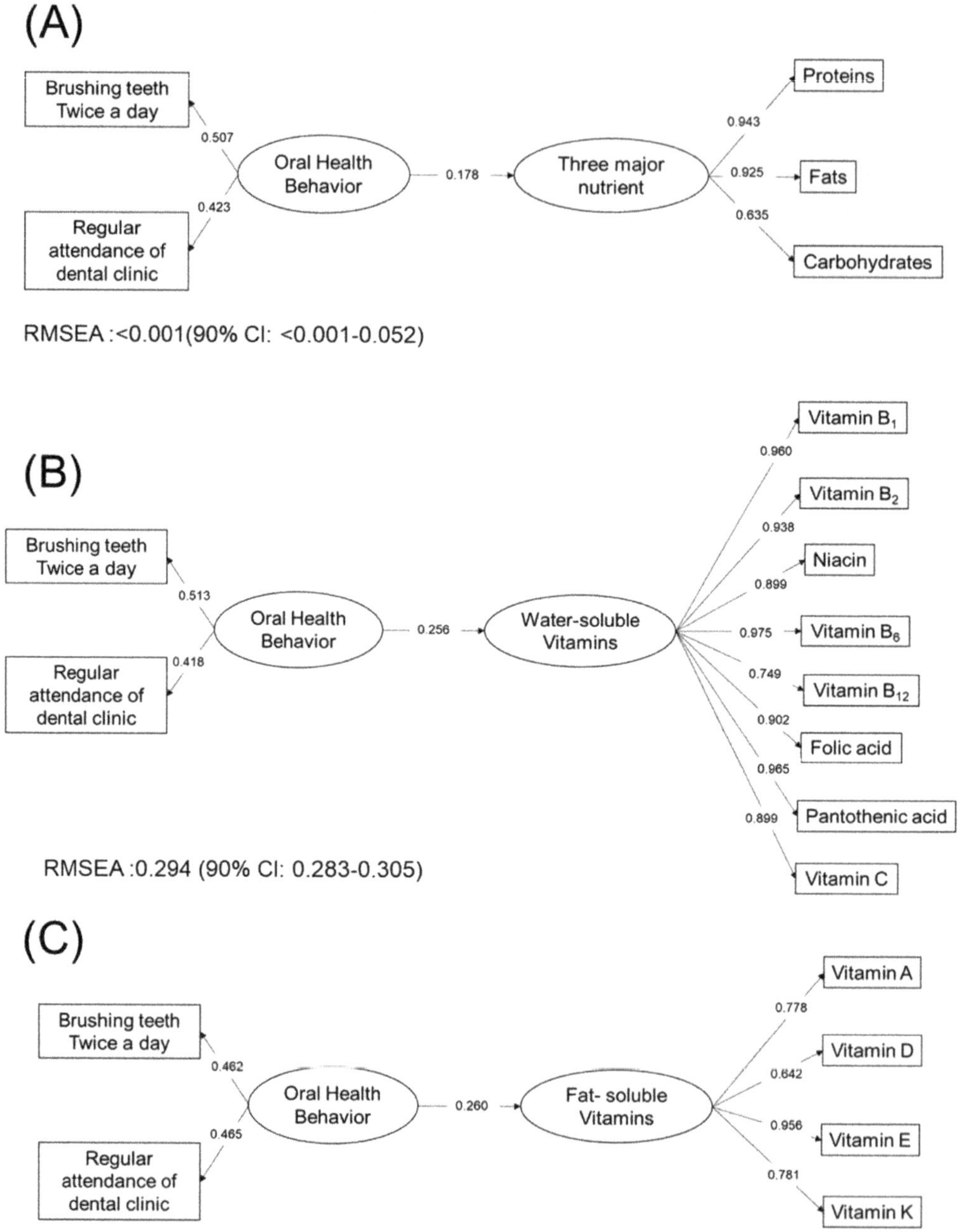

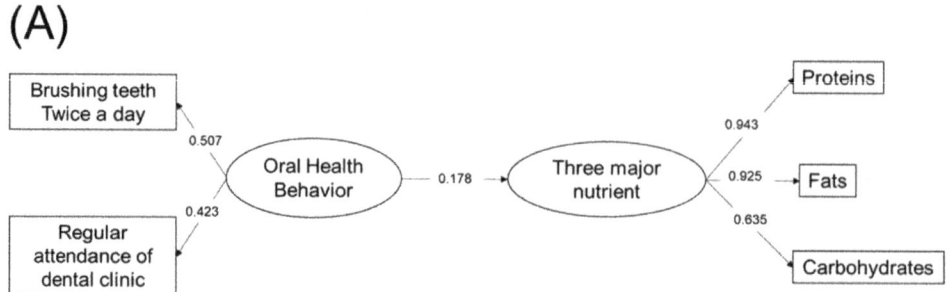

Figure 3. Cont.

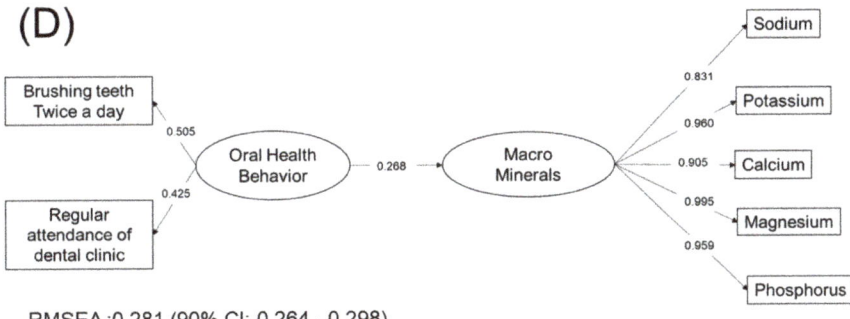

RMSEA :0.281 (90% CI: 0.264 - 0.298)

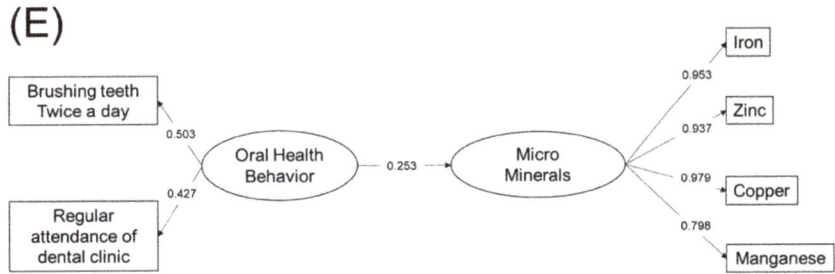

RMSEA :0.132 (90% CI: 0.110 - 0.155)

Figure 3. Structural equation modeling of oral health behavior and nutrition intakes: (**A**) three macronutrients; (**B**) water-soluble Vitamins; (**C**) fat-soluble vitamins; (**D**) macro minerals; and (**E**) micro minerals.

4. Discussion

In this study, we performed a community-based nutritional survey and investigated the relationship among the nutritional intakes, self-assessed oral function, oral health behavior, and number of teeth. The representativeness of study population was compared with the national survey of Japan. Energy intakes of fats and carbohydrates in men were lower than those of the national survey. It indicated that this study population consisted of healthier men.

Consistent nutrition guidelines are essential to improve health. By using the reference values proposed by Dietary Reference Intakes for Japanese [20,21], nutritional status could be clearly categorized for deficiency. Subjects investigated in this study were independent subjects more than 50 years old. Some of the nutrient intakes were not sufficient. Around 90% of subjects had excess salts.

A previous community-based study carried out in Hungary concluded that, for vitamins, the intakes of vitamin B_1, B_2, B_6, B_{12}, niacin, and vitamin C are in line with the recommendations [28]. Vitamin D and folic acid intakes are critically low, particularly in the elderly. In this study, 97.9% of subjects' intake of vitamin B_{12} for EAR was sufficient, while 71.0% for vitamin B_2 and 62.2% for vitamin B_6. However, only 35.5% of subjects consumed sufficient vitamin B_1 for EAR. In contrast, 91.6% of subjects' intakes of vitamin D for AI were sufficient. Japanese food often uses fish as main dish. These foods are rich in vitamin D. For macro minerals, another study showed that the intakes of iron, copper, and manganese compared with the recommendations were insufficient [29]. In this study, the percentages of subjects with sufficient intakes of iron and copper for ERA were 80% and 86.4%, respectively. In contrast, for manganese, the percentage of sufficient subjects' intakes was only 40.2%.

The oral frailty screening questionnaire consisted of eight items. Items concerned self-assessed oral functions, daily activity, and oral health behavior. The items concerning self-assessed oral function and daily activity showed almost no significant correlation with nutrition intakes. In addition, the number of remaining teeth had almost no significant correlation with nutrition intakes. In contrast, two items concerning oral health behavior, namely brushing teeth twice a day and regular attendance of dental clinic, had significant correlation with intakes of most of the nutrients. In this study, nutrients intake status was correlated with oral health behavior but not oral functions and number of remaining teeth.

Several studies have shown that oral functions and number of remaining teeth have statistically significant correlation with the mortality of older adults [10]. However, the number of remaining teeth was conflicting. In contrast, oral functions, especially masticatory function, can be the predicator for mortality. A study has shown that oral function and serum levels albumin, which represent the nutritional status, affect mortality independently [10]. In this study, nutritional status had correlation with oral health behavior, which reflects health literacy.

By the structural equation modeling shown in Figure 3, the coefficients of brushing twice a day were larger than those of regular attendance of dental clinic, indicating that the nutritional intake was dependent on daily health behavior rather than attendance of dental clinic. As primary healthcare, dental clinic has an important role in health promotion. Dental clinic provides treatment with holistic, contentious stance. It should lead to behavior modification [30].

Self-assessed oral function and number of remaining teeth had almost no correlation with the nutritional intakes. Masticatory functions contribute to food digestion and it expands the food choice. Therefore, it can lead to the variation of food and in turn to the improvement of nutritional status. However, food preference or food choice may be robust, and they may not easily change. Therefore, nutritional instruction after oral rehabilitation is necessary. It also plays an important role in the primary healthcare of dentistry.

There are several limitations of this study. The study design is cross sectional. A longitudinal study is necessary to investigate the changes of health status. Information on oral status was limited to the number of remaining teeth. Other oral conditions such as dental caries and periodontal status should be investigated. The oral functions and nutritional intakes investigated in this study were self-assessed. Measuring devices for oral function are available. More precise and objective data on oral function are necessary. Health status other than BMI should be measured. However, overcoming these limitations requires time and resources. This study applied simplified methods to collect larger sample size for the robustness of the data. Propagation of oral frailty has just started in Japan. This study is the first that investigated oral frailty and nutritional intakes. In Japan, the government presents optimal nutritional values by gender and age groups. It is important to evaluate the nutritional intakes of the optimal values by gender, age, and race.

Recovering oral functions by prosthodontic treatment cannot change the nutritional status. In addition to prosthodontic treatment, nutritional instructions are effective to improve nutritional status [31]. Dental clinic is a suitable place for the nutritional instructions along with recovering and maintaining oral functions [32].

In conclusion, comprehensive health instructions including nutrition and oral health education are necessary for health promotion.

Supplementary Materials: The following are available online at http://www.mdpi.com/2072-6643/12/9/2886/s1, Figure S1: Scatter plot of BMI against proportion of energy by three major nutrients. Figure S2: Number of subjects against sum of sufficient nutrition. Table S1: Comparison with Japanese national health and nutritional survey. Table S2: Difference of number of remaining teeth by BMI and three macronutrients. Table S3: Cross tabulation by nutrition intakes against items of oral frail questionnaire. Table S4: Mean and median values of nutrition intakes against items of oral frail questionnaire.

Author Contributions: Conceptualization, Y.N., Y.I. (Yoshimasa Ishii), S.S. (Shunsuke Suzuki), K.M., A.S., S.S. (Senichi Suzuki), J.T., Y.I. (Yasuo Ishiwata), K.Y. and Y.C.; methodology, Y.N., Y.I. (Yoshimasa Ishii), S.S. (Shunsuke Suzuki), K.M., A.S., S.S. (Senichi Suzuki), J.T., Y.I. (Yoshimasa Ishii), K.Y. and Y.C.; software, Y.N.; validation, Y.N. and Y.I. (Yoshimasa Ishii); formal analysis, Y.N.; investigation, Y.I. (Yasuo Ishiwata), S.S. (Shunsuke

Suzuki), K.M., A.S., S.S. (Senichi Suzuki), J.T., Y.I. (Yasuo Ishiwata), K.Y. and Y.C.; data curation, M.I., K.S., E.K., A.O. and R.O.; writing—original draft preparation, Y.N.; writing—review and editing, Y.N.; visualization, Y.N.; project administration, Y.N., Y.I. (Yoshimasa Ishii), S.S. (Shunsuke Suzuki), K.M., A.S., S.S. (Senichi Suzuki), J.T., Y.I. (Yasuo Ishiwata), K.Y. and Y.C.; and funding acquisition, S.S. (Senichi Suzuki), Y.I. (Yasuo Ishiwata) and N.H. All authors have read and agreed to the published version of the manuscript.

Funding: This research was funded by Annual budget of Ebina city for health promotion.

Acknowledgments: We thank Masaru Uchino, Mayor of Ebina city for adopting this project as a health promotion policy plan of Ebina city and supporting funds.

Conflicts of Interest: The authors declare no conflict of interest.

References

1. Hirschfeld, J.; Higham, J.; Chatzistavrianou, D.; Blair, F.; Richards, A.; Chapple, I.L.C. Systemic disease or periodontal disease? Distinguishing causes of gingival inflammation: A guide for dental practitioners. Part 1: Immune-Mediated, autoinflammatory, and hereditary lesions. *Br. Dent. J.* **2019**, *227*, 961–966. [CrossRef] [PubMed]
2. Hirschfeld, J.; Higham, J.; Blair, F.; Richards, A.; Chapple, I.L.C. Systemic disease or periodontal disease? Distinguishing causes of gingival inflammation: A guide for dental practitioners. Part 2: Cancer related, infective, and other causes of gingival pathology. *Br. Dent J.* **2019**, *227*, 1029–1034. [CrossRef] [PubMed]
3. Ahn-Jarvis, J.H.; Piancino, M.G. Chapter 14: Impact of Oral Health on Diet/Nutrition. *Monogr. Oral. Sci.* **2020**, *28*, 134–147. [CrossRef] [PubMed]
4. Ritchie, C.S.; Joshipura, K.; Hung, H.C.; Douglass, C.W. Nutrition as a mediator in the relation between oral and systemic disease: Associations between specific measures of adult oral health and nutrition outcomes. *Crit. Rev. Oral. Biol. Med.* **2002**, *13*, 291–300. [CrossRef] [PubMed]
5. Shwe, P.S.; Ward, S.; Thein, P.M.; Junckerstorff, R. Frailty, oral health and nutrition in geriatrics inpatients: A cross-sectional study. *Gerodontology* **2019**, *36*, 223–228. [CrossRef] [PubMed]
6. N'gom, P.I.; Woda, A.A. Influence of impaired mastication on nutrition. *J. Prosthet. Dent.* **2002**, *87*, 667–673. [CrossRef] [PubMed]
7. Hollis, J.H. The effect of mastication on food intake, satiety and body weight. *Physiol. Behav.* **2018**, *193*, 242–245. [CrossRef] [PubMed]
8. Okamoto, N.; Amano, N.; Nakamura, T.; Yanagi, M. Relationship between tooth loss, low masticatory ability, and nutritional indices in the elderly: A cross-sectional study. *BMC Oral Health* **2019**, *19*, 110. [CrossRef] [PubMed]
9. Horibe, Y.; Ueda, T.; Watanabe, Y.; Motokawa, K.; Edahiro, A.; Hirano, H.; Shirobe, M.; Ogami, K.; Kawai, H.; Obuchi, S.; et al. A 2-year longitudinal study of the relationship between masticatory function and progression to frailty or pre-frailty among community-dwelling Japanese aged 65 and older. *J. Oral. Rehabil.* **2018**, *45*, 864–870. [CrossRef] [PubMed]
10. Nomura, Y.; Kakuta, E.; Okada, A.; Otsuka, R.; Shimada, M.; Tomizawa, Y.; Taguchi, C.; Arikawa, K.; Daikoku, H.; Sato, T.; et al. Effects of self-assessed chewing ability, tooth loss and serum albumin on mortality in 80-year-old individuals: A 20-year follow-up study. *BMC Oral Health* **2020**, *20*, 122. [CrossRef] [PubMed]
11. Wright, F.A.C.; Law, G.G.; Milledge, K.L.; Chu, S.K.; Hsu, B.; Valdez, E.; Naganathan, V.; Hirani, V.; Blyth, F.M.; LeCouteur, D.G.; et al. Chewing function, general health and the dentition of older Australian men: The Concord Health and Ageing in Men Project. *Community Dent. Oral. Epidemiol.* **2019**, *47*, 134–141. [CrossRef] [PubMed]
12. Tanaka, T.; Takahashi, K.; Hirano, H.; Kikutani, T.; Watanabe, Y.; Ohara, Y.; Furuya, H.; Tetsuo, T.; Akishita, M.; Iijima, K. Oral Frailty as a Risk Factor for Physical Frailty and Mortality in Community-Dwelling Elderly. *J. Gerontol. A Biol. Sci. Med. Sci.* **2018**, *73*, 1661–1667. [CrossRef] [PubMed]
13. Kera, T.; Kawai, H.; Yoshida, H.; Hirano, H.; Kojima, M.; Fujiwara, Y.; Ihara, K.; Obuchi, S. Classification of frailty using the Kihon checklist: A cluster analysis of older adults in urban areas. *Geriatr. Gerontol. Int.* **2017**, *17*, 69–77. [CrossRef] [PubMed]
14. World Health Organization. Guideline: Sugars Intake for Adults and Children 2015. Available online: https://www.who.int/publications/i/item/9789241549028 (accessed on 1 September 2020).

15. Valenzuela, M.J.; Waterhouse, B.; Aggarwal, V.R.; Bloor, K.; Doran, T. Effect of sugar-sweetened beverages on oral health: A systematic review and meta-analysis. *Eur. J. Public Health* **2020**, ckaa147. [CrossRef] [PubMed]
16. von Philipsborn, P.; Stratil, J.M.; Burns, J.; Busert, L.K.; Pfandenhauer, L.M.; Polus, S.; Holzapfel, C.; Hauner, H.; Rehfuess, E.A. Environmental Interventions to Reduce the Consumption of Sugar-Sweetened Beverages: Abridged Cochrane Systematic Review. *Obes Facts.* **2020**, *12*, 1–21. [CrossRef] [PubMed]
17. O'Connor, J.L.P.; Milledge, K.L.; O'Leary, F.; Cumming, R.; Eberhard, J.; Hirani, V. Poor dietary intake of nutrients and food groups are associated with increased risk of periodontal disease among community-dwelling older adults: A systematic literature review. *Nutr. Rev.* **2020**, *78*, 175–188. [CrossRef] [PubMed]
18. Tenelanda-López, D.; Valdivia-Moral, P.; Castro-Sánchez, M. Eating Habits and Their Relationship to Oral Health. *Nutrients* **2020**, *12*, 2619. [CrossRef] [PubMed]
19. Costacurta, M.; DiRenzo, L.; Sicuro, L.; Gratteri, S.; Lorenzo, A.D.; Docimo, R. Dental caries and childhood obesity: Analysis of food intakes, lifestyle. *Eur. J. Paediatr. Dent.* **2014**, *15*, 343–348. [PubMed]
20. Ministry of Health, Labor and Welfare. Overview of Dietary Reference Intakes for Japanese (2015). Available online: https://www.mhlw.go.jp/file/06-Seisakujouhou-10900000-Kenkoukyoku/Overview.pdf (accessed on 1 September 2020).
21. Ministry of Health, Labor and Welfare. Overview of Dietary Reference Intakes for Japanese (2020). Available online: https://www.mhlw.go.jp/content/10904750/000586553.pdf (accessed on 1 September 2020).
22. Kobayashi, S.; Murakami, K.; Sasaki, S.; Okubo, H.; Hirota, N.; Notsu, A.; Fukui, M.; Date, C. Comparison of relative validity of food group intakes estimated by comprehensive and brief-type self-administered diet history questionnaires against 16 d dietary records in Japanese adults. *Public Health Nutr.* **2011**, *14*, 1200–1211. [CrossRef] [PubMed]
23. Kobayashi, S.; Honda, S.; Murakami, K.; Sasaki, S.; Okubo, H.; Hirota, N.; Notsu, A.; Fukui, M.; Date, C. Both comprehensive and brief self-administered diet history questionnaires satisfactorily rank nutrient intakes in Japanese adults. *J. Epidemiol.* **2012**, *22*, 151–159. [CrossRef] [PubMed]
24. Maruyama, K.; Kokubo, Y.; Yamanaka, T.; Watanabe, M.; Iso, H.; Okamura, T.; Miyamoto, Y. The reasonable reliability of a self-administered food frequency questionnaire for an urban, Japanese, middle-aged population: The Suita study. *Nutr. Res.* **2015**, *35*, 14–22. [CrossRef] [PubMed]
25. Kobayashi, S.; Yuan, X.; Sasaki, S.; Osawa, Y.; Hirata, T.; Abe, Y.; Takayama, M.; Arai, Y.; Masui, Y.; Ishizaki, T. Relative validity of brief-type self-administered diet history questionnaire among very old Japanese aged 80 years or older. *Public Health Nutr.* **2019**, *22*, 212–222. [CrossRef] [PubMed]
26. Nordenram, G.; Ryd-Kjellen, E.; Johansson, G.; Nordstrom, G.; Winblad, B. Alzheimer's disease, oral function and nutritional status. *Gerodontology* **1996**, *13*, 9–16. [CrossRef] [PubMed]
27. Ministry of Health, Labor and Welfare. National Health and Nutrition Examination Survey (2018). Available online: https://www.mhlw.go.jp/stf/newpage_08789.html (accessed on 1 September 2020).
28. Molnár, E.S.; Nagy-Lőrincz, Z.; Nagy, B.; Bakacs, M.; Kis, O.; Nagy, E.S.; Martos, É. Hungarian Diet and Nutritional Status Survey—The OTAP2014 study. V. Vitamin intake of the Hungarian population. *Orv. Hetil.* **2017**, *158*, 1302–1313. [CrossRef] [PubMed]
29. Nagy, B.; Nagy-Lőrincz, Z.; Bakacs, M.; Illés, É.; Nagy, E.S.; Martos, É. Hungarian Diet and Nutritional Status Survey—OTÁP2014. III. Macroelement intake of the Hungarian population]. *Orv. Hetil.* **2017**, *158*, 653–661. [CrossRef] [PubMed]
30. Brandstetter, S.; Rüter, J.; Curbach, J.; Loss, J. A systematic review on empowerment for healthy nutrition in health promotion. *Public Health Nutr.* **2015**, *18*, 3146–3154. [CrossRef] [PubMed]
31. Takeuchi, H.; Terada, M.; Kobayashi, K.; Uraguchi, M.; Nomura, Y.; Hanada, N. Influences of Masticatory Function Recovery Combined with Health Guidance on Body Composition and Metabolic Parameters. *Open Dent. J.* **2019**, *13*, 124–136. [CrossRef]
32. Nomura, Y.; Takeuchi, H.; Shigemoto, S.; Okada, A.; Shigeta, Y.; Ogawa, T.; Hanada, N. Secondary Endpoint of the Prosthodontics. *Int. J. Clin. Case Stud.* **2017**, *3*, IJCCS-117. [CrossRef]

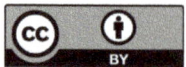

© 2020 by the authors. Licensee MDPI, Basel, Switzerland. This article is an open access article distributed under the terms and conditions of the Creative Commons Attribution (CC BY) license (http://creativecommons.org/licenses/by/4.0/).

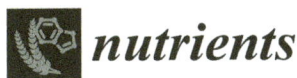

Article

Breakfast Consumption in Low-Income Hispanic Elementary School-Aged Children: Associations with Anthropometric, Metabolic, and Dietary Parameters

Matthew R. Jeans [1,*], Fiona M. Asigbee [1], Matthew J. Landry [1], Sarvenaz Vandyousefi [1], Reem Ghaddar [1], Heather J. Leidy [1,2] and Jaimie N. Davis [1]

1. The University of Texas at Austin, Department of Nutritional Sciences, 200 W 24th Street, Stop A2700, Austin, TX 78712, USA; fiona.asigbee@utexas.edu (F.M.A.); matthewlandry@utexas.edu (M.J.L.); sarvenaz.vandyousefi@nyulangone.org (S.V.); reemghaddar94@gmail.com (R.G.); heather.leidy@austin.utexas.edu (H.J.L.); jaimie.davis@austin.utexas.edu (J.N.D.)
2. Department of Pediatrics, Dell Medical Center, The University of Texas at Austin, 1400 Barbara Jordan Blvd, Austin, TX 78723, USA
* Correspondence: mjeans@utexas.edu; Tel.: +1-931-625-5969

Received: 19 May 2020; Accepted: 6 July 2020; Published: 9 July 2020

Abstract: Breakfast consumption is associated with lower obesity prevalence and cardiometabolic risk and higher dietary quality (DQ) in children. Low-income, Hispanic populations are disproportionately affected by obesity and cardiometabolic risks. This study examined the relationship between breakfast consumption groups (BCG) on anthropometric, metabolic, and dietary parameters in predominately low-income, Hispanic children from 16 Texas schools. Cross-sectional data were from TX Sprouts, a school-based gardening, nutrition, and cooking randomized controlled trial. Anthropometric measurements included height, weight, body mass index, body fat percent via bioelectrical impedance, waist circumference, and blood pressure. Metabolic parameters included fasting plasma glucose, insulin, glycated hemoglobin, cholesterol, and triglycerides. DQ and BCG were assessed via two 24-h dietary recalls. Multivariate multiple regression examined relationships between BCG and anthropometric, metabolic, and dietary parameters. This study included 671 students (mean age 9 years, 58% Hispanic, 54% female, 66% free/reduced lunch, 17% breakfast skippers). No relationships were observed between BCG and anthropometric or metabolic parameters. BCG had higher DQ; higher daily protein, total sugar, and added sugar intake; and lower daily fat intake. Skipping breakfast was associated with lower DQ; higher daily fat intake; and lower daily protein intake. Longitudinal research examining breakfast quality on cardiometabolic outcomes in low-income, Hispanic children is warranted.

Keywords: breakfast consumption; breakfast composition; children; dietary intake; dietary quality; diet patterns; cardiometabolic outcomes; adiposity

1. Introduction

Obesity prevalence has nearly tripled since 1975, affecting 18.5% of children and adolescents in the U.S., with those of Hispanic origin disproportionately affected at 25.8% [1]. Breakfast consumption has been a target of ongoing research in both predicting and preventing overweight and obesity prevalence [2]. Metabolic and physiological benefits of breakfast consumption in children include improved lipid panels, glucose control, and blood pressure and decreased fasting insulin [3–6]. Breakfast consumption is associated with lower cardiometabolic risks [2], including dyslipidemia [7], and lower metabolic syndrome risk in children [4,5,8,9]. However, few studies have evaluated breakfast consumption on cardiometabolic risks in primarily low-income, Hispanic children.

Despite breakfast consumption being associated with improved health outcomes in children and adolescents [5,10–18], the International Breakfast Research Initiative reports that only one third to one half of older children (11–15 years of age) consume breakfast every day [19]. In addition, the prevalence of skipping breakfast has been shown to increase with age [20]. Children and adolescents skip breakfast more than any other meal [21,22], with one study showing higher prevalence of skipping in Hispanic youth (32%) when compared to Caucasian youth (19%) [22]. Primary reasons for skipping breakfast include financial constraints and having inaccessibility to appropriate breakfast foods [23]. Hispanic households have higher prevalence of food insecurity, which has been associated with increased obesity prevalence in Hispanic children [24,25]. Nonetheless, while evidence supports the daily consumption of breakfast, studies have found conflicting results to substantiate this evidence. Some studies have shown a null association between breakfast consumption and weight management while others have found a positive association [26–30]. Potential reasons for the conflicting findings could be attributed to the quality of foods consumed at breakfast and/or the influence of breakfast on the overall diet.

Breakfast consumption is associated with meeting dietary intake recommendations and having superior overall diet quality in children [5,31,32]. Independent of breakfast consumption, breakfast composition has been associated with varied dietary quality [31,33]. Measures of dietary quality included evaluation of micronutrients, specifically shortfall nutrients (i.e., vitamin E, calcium, magnesium, iron, and zinc), and use of the Nutrient Rich Foods Index and the USDA Healthy Eating Index 2015 (HEI-2015) [31–33]. While associated with higher overall diet quality, regular breakfast consumers display higher intakes of saturated fats [5], sweets [33], and flavored milk [33] at breakfast, potentially eliciting a negative effect on adiposity and weight management. These counterintuitive findings could be due to fortification of common breakfast foods (i.e., cereals, nutrition bars, etc.) that tend to be high in saturated fats and added sugars, while still providing vitamins and minerals that contribute to diet quality. Furthermore, Deshmukh-Taskar et al. posed that consumption of milk at breakfast contributed to increased calcium intake [31]. Similar to flavored milk, this could explain why higher overall diet quality is observed, regardless of its other negative qualities.

These inconsistencies highlight the complex interaction between breakfast consumption and body weight, metabolism, and dietary habits. The evaluation of breakfast consumption is limited in primarily low-income and Hispanic populations, especially children. This study aims to (1) assess the relationship between breakfast consumption (skipping, intermittent consumption, and regular consumption) on anthropometric and metabolic parameters; (2) assess the relationship between breakfast consumption on daily dietary intake; and (3) assess the relationship between varied breakfast consumption patterns (intermittent vs. regular) on breakfast dietary intake in primarily low-income, Hispanic elementary school-aged children. It was hypothesized that breakfast consumption would be related to lower cardiometabolic risks and higher daily dietary quality, and that regular breakfast consumption would be related to a higher-quality breakfast meal than intermittent breakfast consumption.

2. Materials and Methods

2.1. Study Design

This cross-sectional study used baseline data from TX Sprouts, a school-based cluster randomized controlled gardening, nutrition, and cooking intervention. The study design for the TX Sprouts intervention has been described in detail elsewhere [34]. TX Sprouts recruited 3rd–5th grade students and their parents from 16 elementary schools in the Greater Austin, TX, area. All schools had to meet the following inclusion criteria: (1) high proportion of Hispanic children (>50%); (2) high proportion of children enrolled in the free and reduced lunch (FRL) program (>50%); (3) location within 60 miles of the University of Texas at Austin campus; and (4) no pre-existing school garden or gardening program. The first 16 schools that met criteria and agreed to participate were randomly assigned to receive the intervention (n = 8 schools) or delayed intervention (n = 8 schools), serving as the control group. This trial was registered at ClinicalTrials.gov (NCT02668744).

2.2. Study Population

There was a total of 3302 students who obtained parental consent to participate in TX Sprouts. Of those, clinical data was collected on 3135. Sixteen students (eight male and eight female) were randomly selected from each grade level at each school to be contacted for recalls ($n = 48$/school). If any of the 16 originally selected students were unavailable or did not want to participate in recalls, then additional students were randomly selected to take their place. Dietary recalls were collected on a total subsample of 783 children—of which 23 had completed only one 24-h recall and were thus omitted. An additional child was omitted due to the breakfast energy cut point leaving only one day of recalls thereafter. Students were excluded from analyses for missing anthropometric data ($n = 32$) and demographic data ($n = 56$). In addition, one student was omitted due to the breakfast energy cut point. The total analytical sample was 671 students. Figure 1 provides a detailed consort diagram showing participant flow through the study.

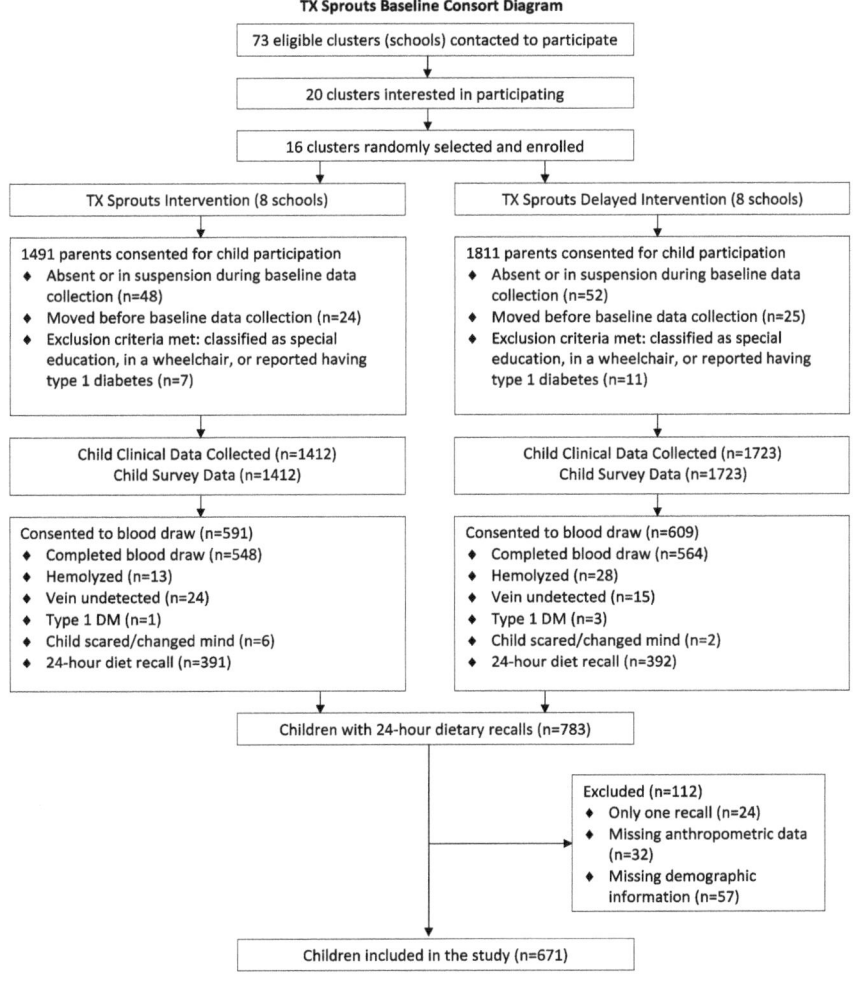

Figure 1. Consort diagram.

2.3. Recruitment

All 3rd–5th grade students and parents of the recruited schools were contacted to participate via information tables at "Back to School" and "Meet the Teacher" events, flyers sent home with students, and classroom announcements made by teachers. Recruitment materials were available in both English and Spanish. Both parental consent and student assent were required for inclusion in the study. The study was conducted in accordance with the Declaration of Helsinki, and all procedures pertaining to human subjects were approved by the Institutional Review Boards of the University of Texas at Austin (IRB#2014-11-0045) and all associated school district review boards.

2.4. Anthropometric Parameters

Height was measured using a free-standing stadiometer to the nearest 0.1 cm (Seca, Birmingham, UK). In a private screening area, participants were asked to gather clothing above the waist so that waist circumference could be measured over skin using the National Health and Nutrition Examination Survey (NHANES) protocol [35]. Participants were asked to remove all footwear and heavy and/or layered clothing to obtain weight and bioelectrical impedance, which were assessed with a Tanita Body Fat Analyzer (Tanita Corporation of America Inc., IL, USA, model TBF 300) that was calibrated to −0.2 kg to account for clothing remaining. BMI z-scores were determined using Centers for Disease Control and Prevention (CDC) age- and gender-specific values [36]. Blood pressure was measured via an automated monitor (Omron, Schaumberg, IL, USA) with a child cuff or, in some cases, an adult cuff, which was used when the child cuff did not properly fit to provide an accurate reading.

2.5. Metabolic Parameters

Optional fasting blood draws were collected before the school day between 6:00 a.m. and 7:00 a.m. on a subsample of students at baseline. Those who opted to not participate in the blood draw were still able to participate in all other TX Sprouts evaluations and activities. Eligible students and their families received flyers and text message reminders about the optional blood draws and to come in fasting, having nothing to eat or drink other than water after midnight. Blood samples were collected by certified phlebotomists or nurses with experience drawing blood in children with obesity and were conducted in a private room at the schools. Students received a $20 incentive for participation in the blood draw. Samples were collected on site and transported on ice to the University of Texas at Austin laboratory.

Directly following collection, whole blood was placed on ice and transferred to the laboratory on the University of Texas at Austin campus, where it was spun and Clinical Laboratory Improvement Amendments (CLIA) certified glucose using HemoCue Glucose 201 (HemoCue America, Brea, CA, USA). Due to a larger than expected proportion of students having prediabetes using the American Diabetes Association definition (fasting plasma glucose of 100–125 mg/dL or HbA1c of 5.7–6.4%) [37], HbA1c measurement was added in the last two waves, explaining the lower number of samples and values observed for HbA1c. HbA1c assays using DCA Vantage Analyzer (Siemens Medical Solutions, Malvern, PA, USA) were performed on whole blood. Remaining blood was centrifuged, aliquoted, and stored at −80 °C. Samples were transported on dry ice to Baylor University for assessment of insulin, cholesterol, and triglycerides. Insulin was evaluated using an automated enzyme immunoassay system analyzer (Tosoh Bioscience, Inc. San Francisco, CA, USA). Total cholesterol, high-density lipoprotein (HDL), and triglyceride levels were measured using Vitros chemistry DT slides (Ortho Clinical Diagnostics Inc., Rochester, NY, USA); low-density lipoprotein (LDL) was calculated using the Friedwald equation [38].

2.6. Dietary Parameters

Dietary intake was collected using a validated two 24-h dietary recall method on a random subsample of children at baseline [39]. Recalls were collected via telephone by trained staff and supervised by a Registered Dietitian Nutritionist using Nutrition Data System for Research (NDS-R, 2016 version), a computer-based software application that facilitates the collection of recalls in a standardized fashion [40]. NDS-R generated nutrient and food/beverage servings and groupings, and HEI-2015 scores were calculated to assess dietary quality [41–44]. The HEI-2015 is composed of thirteen food components representative of the dietary recommendations based on the *Dietary Guidelines for Americans, 2015–2020*. These HEI-2015 components are divided into two groups: nine adequacy components (i.e., greens and beans, total fruits and vegetables, whole fruits, dairy, while grains, total protein foods, seafood and plant proteins, and fatty acids) and four moderation components (i.e., sodium, added sugars, refined grains, and saturated fat). Higher adequacy component scores are indicative of higher intake while higher moderation component scores are indicative of lower intake. The individual component scores are summed to an overall total HEI-2015 score ranging from 0 to 100. Higher HEI-2015 scores indicate higher dietary quality, per the *Dietary Guidelines for Americans, 2015–2020*.

Dietary intake data gathered by interview were governed by a multiple-pass interview approach [45]. Prior to the dietary recalls, Food Amounts Booklets, developed by the Nutrition Coordinating Center (NCC), were distributed to and sent home with the students. The booklets were provided in both English and Spanish and contained pictures of serving sizes to assist students in estimating serving sizes of foods and beverages reported during the dietary recall. Parents and/or guardians were allowed to assist with information regarding food items and portion sizes when needed. Students received a $10 incentive upon completion of both 24-h dietary recalls. Quality assurance was conducted on all dietary recall data by additional trained research staff. All daily dietary parameters were averages over the two days dietary recalls were conducted.

2.7. Breakfast Parameters

During each 24-h dietary recall, students were asked to name each eating occasion (EO) and the time of day when the EO occurred. Response options included: breakfast, brunch, lunch, dinner/supper, snack, beverage only, school lunch, or other. Dietary values were averaged across the two days of recall information to obtain mean values of consumption. Students were classified as breakfast consumers if they referred to an EO as "breakfast" and the energy intake was at least 15% of total daily energy and consumption occurred before 10:00 a.m. These criteria have been shown as an appropriate method for defining a breakfast meal [46–49]. If two breakfasts were consumed on the same day before 10:00 a.m. (i.e., one from home and one from school), then dietary values were combined before averaging with the second dietary recall.

In line with previous work evaluating breakfast consumption [31,50–52], breakfast consumption groups (BCG) were defined using the dietary recall data: (1) SKIPPERS, having no breakfast EO on either recall day; (2) INTERMITTENT, having a breakfast EO on only one recall day; and (3) REGULAR, having a breakfast EO on both recall days. As a result, breakfast dietary parameters for intermittent consumers were representative of intake for one day, while breakfast dietary parameters for regular consumers were representative of the average intake over two days.

2.8. Statistical Analysis

Data were examined for normality, and transformations were made if data deviated from normality. All variables were transformed for normality except BMI z-score, fasting plasma glucose, total cholesterol (mg/dL), non-HDL cholesterol (mg/dL), LDL cholesterol (mg/dL), HEI-2015 scores, carbohydrate (% kcal), fat (% kcal), total sugar (% kcal), and breakfast total sugar (% kcal). The negative reciprocal method was used for HbA1c (%) and diastolic BP (mmHg). The square root method was used for added sugar (% kcal), breakfast protein (% kcal), breakfast fat (% kcal), breakfast added sugar (% kcal), and whole grains (serving/day). The cubed method was used for BMI percentile (%). All other variables were log transformed. All analyses were performed using Stata version 16.0 (StataCorp, College Station, TX, USA), and the significance was set at $p < 0.05$.

Multivariate multiple regression assessed relationships between anthropometric and metabolic parameters by breakfast consumption groups. For anthropometric parameters, the model included waist circumference, percent body fat, BMI z-score, systolic blood pressure, and diastolic blood pressure. For metabolic parameters, one multivariate model included fasting glucose, insulin, total cholesterol, and triglycerides, and a second multivariate model included fasting glucose, insulin, HDL, non-HDL, LDL, and triglycerides. Since HbA1c was assessed only in the last two waves of the intervention, it was assessed in a third multivariate model including fasting glucose, total cholesterol, and triglycerides. All multivariate models pertaining to metabolic outcomes adjusted for age, sex, race/ethnicity, free and reduced lunch status, total energy, and BMI z-score (only in metabolic models).

Multivariate multiple regression assessed relationships between daily dietary parameters by breakfast consumption groups. Daily eating occasions, HEI-2015 scores, and total energy were assessed in univariate models. For daily nutrient intake, one multivariate model included percent protein, percent fat, percent carbohydrate, total fiber, and percent total sugar, and a second multivariate model included percent protein, percent fat, percent carbohydrate, soluble fiber, insoluble fiber, and percent added sugar. For daily food servings, one multivariate model included vegetables (including 100% juice and potatoes), fruit (including 100% juice), dairy (including flavored milk), SSBs (including flavored milk), whole grains, refined grains, meats, and legumes. A second multivariate model included vegetables (excluding 100% juice), fruit (excluding 100% juice), dairy (excluding flavored milk), SSBs (excluding flavored milk), whole grains, refined grains, meats, and legumes. A third multivariate model was the same as the second multivariate model but replaced vegetables (excluding 100% juice) with vegetables (excluding 100% juice and potatoes). All multivariate models pertaining to daily dietary parameters adjusted for age, sex, race/ethnicity, free and reduced lunch status, BMI z-score, day of the week, and total energy.

Multivariate multiple regression assessed relationships between breakfast composition between intermittent and regular consumers. Breakfast energy was assessed in a univariate model, adjusting for subsequent energy. For breakfast nutrient intake, one multivariate model included breakfast percent protein, percent fat, percent carbohydrate, total fiber, and percent total sugar, and a second multivariate model included breakfast percent protein, percent fat, percent carbohydrate, soluble fiber, insoluble fiber, and percent added sugar. For breakfast food servings, the multivariate model included breakfast whole and refined grain servings. All multivariate models pertaining to breakfast composition adjusted for age, sex, race/ethnicity, free and reduced lunch status, BMI z-score, day of the week, and total energy.

3. Results

3.1. Study Sample

The basic demographic, anthropometric, and dietary characteristics data are presented in Tables 1 and 2. The sample was predominately Hispanic (58%) and female (54%), with an average age of 9.3 years. Reported enrollment of children in the Free and Reduced Lunch Program was 66%. The average BMI z-score was 0.8, and nearly 49% of children had overweight or obesity. The prevalence of BCG was 17% for skippers, 37% for intermittent consumers, and 46% for regular consumers. The average dietary quality, represented by the Healthy Eating Index—2015, was 53.8 out of a possible 100.

Table 1. Physical characteristics of the analytic sample ($n = 671$).

Variable	Value [a]
Sex (F)	364 (54.3%)
Age (years)	9.3 (9.2, 9.3)
Ethnicity	
Hispanic	392 (58.4%)
Non-Hispanic	279 (41.6%)
Free/Reduced Lunch	446 (66.5%)
Breakfast Consumption Groups	
Skippers	114 (17.0%)
Intermittent Consumers	249 (37.1%)
Regular Consumers	308 (45.9%)
Height (cm)	138.4 (137.8, 139.1)
Weight (kg)	39.4 (38.5, 40.3)
BMI z-score	0.8 (0.8, 0.9)
BMI categories	
Overweight	129 (19.2%)
Obese	198 (29.5%)

[a] All values are n (%) or mean (95% CI).

Table 2. Dietary characteristics of the analytic sample ($n = 671$).

Variable	Mean [a]	95% CIs
Eating occasions	3.3	(3.3, 3.4)
Healthy Eating Index-2015	53.8	(52.8, 54.7)
Total energy (kcal/day)	1446.2	(1405.1, 1487.3)
Carbohydrate (% kcal)	49.7	(49.0, 50.3)
Protein (% kcal)	16.2	(15.9, 16.5)
Fat (% kcal)	33.3	(32.8, 33.8)
Total fiber (g)	12.1	(11.7, 12.6)
Soluble fiber (g)	3.8	(3.7, 4.0)
Insoluble fiber (g)	8.2	(7.9, 8.5)
Total sugar (% kcal)	20.7	(20.2, 21.3)
Added sugar (% kcal)	10.1	(9.6, 10.5)
Total vegetables (serving/day) [b]	1.7	(1.6, 1.8)
Excluding 100% juice	1.7	(1.6, 1.8)
Excluding 100% juice and potatoes	1.5	(1.4, 1.6)
Total Fruits (serving/day)	1.5	(1.4, 1.7)
Excluding 100% juice	0.9	(0.8, 1.0)
Dairy (serving/day)	1.7	(1.6, 1.8)
Excluding flavored milk	1.5	(1.4, 1.6)
Sugar-sweetened beverages (serving/day)	0.7	(0.7, 0.8)
Excluding flavored milk	0.5	(0.4, 0.6)
Whole grains (serving/day)	1.1	(1.0, 1.2)
Refined grains (serving/day)	4.6	(4.4, 4.9)
Meat (serving/day)	3.7	(3.5, 3.8)
Legumes (serving/day)	0.2	(0.16, 0.23)

[a] Dietary data reflects the average of two days. [b] Servings per day.

3.2. Relationships between Breakfast Consumption and Anthropometric and Metabolic Parameters

The relationships between BCG and anthropometric and metabolic parameters are presented in Table 3. There were no significant relationships between breakfast consumption groups and adiposity and metabolic parameters. A Pearson's chi-square test was conducted to determine if these results could be a result of heterogeneous distributions of overweight and obese children between the BCG; however, the result was insignificant ($p = 0.65$) and showed homogenous distributions of BMI categories between the BCG.

Table 3. Multivariate regression models of anthropometric and metabolic parameters with regular consumers as the referent group.

Variable	Overall † p	Skipper β	Skipper (95% CI)	Skipper p	Intermittent β	Intermittent (95% CI)	Intermittent p
Anthropometric Parameters (n = 671)							
Waist circumference (cm) [a]	0.09	0.59	(−1.98, 3.16)	0.62	2.09	(0.08, 4.10)	0.03
Total body fat (%) [a]	0.39	−0.05	(−1.95, 1.86)	0.76	0.82	(−0.67, 2.31)	0.17
BMI z-score [a]	0.12	0.12	(−0.12, 0.36)	0.33	0.19	(0.01, 0.38)	0.04
Systolic blood pressure (mmHg) [a]	0.58	−0.10	(−2.51, 2.31)	0.99	0.84	(−1.05, 2.73)	0.33
Diastolic blood pressure (mmHg) [a]	0.72	0.63	(−1.46, 2.72)	0.64	0.43	(−1.21, 2.06)	0.43
Metabolic Parameters (n = 344)							
Fasting glucose (mg/dL) [b,c,d]	0.89	0.47	(−2.23, 3.17)	0.73	−0.21	(−2.42, 2.01)	0.85
Insulin (μIU/mL) [b,c,d]	0.67	0.89	(−2.29, 4.08)	0.39	1.26	(−1.35, 3.87)	0.90
Triglycerides (mg/dL) [b,c,d]	0.37	4.14	(−7.46, 15.74)	0.61	−5.98	(−15.49, 3.52)	0.32
Total cholesterol (mg/dL) [b,c,d]	0.95	0.42	(−6.82, 7.66)	0.91	0.93	(−5.00, 6.87)	0.76
HDL (mg/dL) [c]	0.96	−0.30	(−2.95, 2.36)	0.89	−0.31	(−2.49, 1.87)	0.77
Non-HDL (mg/dL) [c]	0.91	0.69	(−5.86, 7.24)	0.84	1.18	(−4.19, 6.54)	0.67
LDL (mg/dL) [c]	0.54	−0.15	(−6.05, 5.74)	0.96	2.45	(−2.38, 7.28)	0.32
HbA1c (%) [d]	0.49	−0.09	(−0.15, 0.09)	0.50	0.04	(−0.06, 0.15)	0.53

Abbreviations: BMI, body mass index; HbA1c, glycolated hemoglobin A1C; HDL, high-density lipoprotein; LDL, low-density lipoprotein. Multivariate regression assessed relationships between anthropometric parameters ($n = 671$) and metabolic parameters ($n = 344$) by breakfast consumption groups. Regular consumers served as the referent group for all analyses. † Overall effect of breakfast consumption groups. [a] Model included waist circumference, total body fat, BMI z-score, and blood pressure. [b] Model included fasting glucose, insulin, total cholesterol, and triglycerides. [c] Model included fasting glucose, insulin, triglycerides, HDL, non-HDL, and LDL. [d] HbA1c was assessed only in the last two waves of the intervention, indicative of the smaller sample size ($n = 237$), so it was assessed in an independent model including fasting glucose, insulin, total cholesterol, and triglycerides. A priori covariates included: age, sex, race/ethnicity, free/reduced lunch status, daily energy, and BMI z-score (for metabolic parameters).

3.3. Relationships between Breakfast Consumption and Daily Dietary Parameters

The relationships between BCG and daily dietary parameters are presented in Table 4. On average, there were fewer eating occasions observed in both SKIPPER and INTERMITTENT than REGULAR ($β = −0.87$ & $β = −0.42$, respectively; both $p < 0.001$). Differences in dietary quality, represented by total HEI-2015 scores, were detected between BCG, with SKIPPER and INTERMITTENT having lower scores than REGULAR ($β = −3.88$ & $β = −2.69$, respectively; both $p < 0.02$). Even with fewer eating occasions, INTERMITTENT had higher total daily energy than REGULAR ($β = 174.73$; $p < 0.001$). Daily macronutrient composition varied between BCG. Daily carbohydrate consumption was lower in SKIPPER and INTERMITTENT compared to REGULAR ($β = −7.28$ & $β = −2.82$, respectively; both $p < 0.001$). SKIPPER and INTERMITTENT had lower daily protein consumption than and REGULAR ($β = −1.46$ & $β = −0.96$, respectively; both $p < 0.001$). Lastly, SKIPPER consumed higher daily fat compared to REGULAR ($β = 2.48$; $p = 0.001$). Total fiber consumption was lower in both SKIPPER and INTERMITTENT than REGULAR ($β = −1.03$ & $β = −0.98$, respectively; both $p < 0.01$). Specifically, SKIPPER and INTERMITTENT had lower soluble fiber consumption than REGULAR ($β = −0.62$ & $β = −0.39$, respectively; both $p < 0.001$). Compared to REGULAR, both SKIPPER and INTERMITTENT had lower consumption of total sugar ($β = −5.91$ & $β = −2.03$, respectively; both $p < 0.01$). However, with added sugar, only SKIPPER had lower consumption than REGULAR ($β = −1.64$; both $p = 0.002$). Daily fruit consumption (including 100% juice) was lower in SKIPPER and INTERMITTENT compared to REGULAR ($β = −0.43$ & $β = −0.24$, respectively; both $p < 0.01$). However, when 100% juice was excluded, this relationship was attenuated. Daily consumption of whole grains was lower in SKIPPER compared to REGULAR ($β = −0.14$; $p < 0.001$).

Table 4. Multivariate regression models of daily nutrient intake and daily food and beverage servings with regular consumers as the referent group ($n = 671$).

Variable	Overall [†]		Skipper			Intermittent		
	p	β	(95% CI)	p	β	(95% CI)	p	
Dietary Intake Parameters								
Eating occasions	<0.001 *	−0.87	(−1.01, −0.73)	<0.001 *	−0.42	(−0.53, −0.30)	<0.001 *	
HEI-2015	0.005 *	−3.88	(−6.52, −1.24)	0.004 *	−2.69	(−4.76, −0.62)	0.01 *	
Total energy (kcal)	0.004 *	111.35	(−5.11, 227.81)	0.14	174.73	(84.25, 265.20)	0.001 *	
Protein (%kcal) [a,b]	<0.001 *	−1.46	(−2.26, −0.66)	<0.001 *	−0.96	(−1.59, −0.34)	0.001 *	
Fat (%kcal) [a,b]	0.005 *	2.48	(1.00, 3.95)	0.001 *	0.90	(−0.25, 2.06)	0.13	
Carbohydrate (%kcal) [a,b]	<0.001 *	−7.28	(−9.10, −5.46)	<0.001 *	−2.82	(−4.24, −1.39)	<0.001 *	
Total fiber (g) [a,b]	0.007 *	−1.03	(−1.97, −0.09)	0.02 *	−0.98	(−1.72, −0.25)	0.004 *	
Total sugar (%kcal) [a,b]	<0.001 *	−5.91	(−7.55, −4.26)	<0.001 *	−2.03	(−3.32, −0.75)	0.002 *	
Soluble fiber (g) [b]	<0.001 *	−0.62	(−0.93, −0.31)	<0.001 *	−0.39	(−0.63, −0.14)	0.001 *	
Insoluble fiber (g) [b]	0.051	−0.46	(−1.23, 0.30)	0.12	−0.61	(−1.21, −0.01)	0.02	
Added sugar (%kcal) [b]	0.003 *	−1.64	(−2.91, −0.37)	0.002 *	0.31	(−0.68, 1.30)	0.81	
Food and Beverage Servings								
Whole grains (serving/day) [c,d,e]	0.002 *	−0.14	(−0.40, 0.13)	0.001 *	−0.05	(−0.26, 0.16)	0.37	
Refined grains (serving/day) [c,d,e]	0.16	−0.21	(−0.69, 0.28)	0.06	−0.27	(−0.65, 0.11)	0.32	
Meats (serving/day) [c,d,e]	0.98	0.17	(−0.30, 0.65)	0.94	0.10	(−0.27, 0.48)	0.88	
Legumes (serving/day) [c,d,e]	0.07	0.10	(0.01, 0.19)	0.02	0.01	(−0.06, 0.08)	0.64	
Vegetables, including 100% juice & potatoes (serving/day) [c]	0.87	−0.001	(−0.26, 0.26)	0.86	−0.09	(−0.29, 0.12)	0.69	
Fruit, including 100% juice (serving/day) [c]	0.001 *	−0.43	(−0.77, −0.08)	0.002 *	−0.24	(−0.51, 0.03)	0.003 *	
Dairy, including flavored milk (serving/day) [c]	0.09	−0.18	(−0.40, 0.03)	0.03	−0.09	(−0.26, 0.08)	0.30	
SSBs, including flavored milk (serving/day) [c]	0.44	−0.09	(−0.28, 0.09)	0.42	0.10	(−0.04, 0.25)	0.52	
Vegetables, excluding 100% juice (serving/day) [d,e]	0.85	0.0004	(−0.26, 0.26)	0.85	−0.09	(−0.26, 0.26)	0.66	
Fruit, excluding 100% juice (serving/day) [d,e]	0.29	−0.10	(−0.40, 0.19)	0.27	−0.05	(−0.28, 0.18)	0.15	
Dairy, excluding flavored milk (serving/day) [d,e]	0.40	−0.07	(−0.28, 0.14)	0.27	−0.09	(−0.28, 1.4)	0.26	
SSBs, excluding flavored milk (serving/day) [d,e]	0.65	0.02	(−0.14, 0.18)	0.61	0.10	(−0.03, 0.22)	0.37	
Vegetables, excluding 100% juice & potatoes (serving/day) [e]	0.57	0.03	(−0.22, 0.28)	0.66	−0.12	(−0.31, 0.07)	0.46	

Abbreviations: HEI, healthy eating index; SSBs, sugar-sweetened beverages. * Indicates a statistically significant value of $p < 0.05$. Multivariate regression assessed relationships between all dietary parameters by breakfast consumption groups ($n = 671$). Regular consumers served as the referent group for all analyses. [†] Overall effect of breakfast consumption groups. Eating occasions, HEI-2015 scores, and total energy were assessed in univariate models. [a] Model included percent protein, percent fat, percent carbohydrate, total fiber, and percent total sugar. [b] Model included percent protein, percent fat, percent carbohydrate, soluble fiber, insoluble fiber, and percent added sugar. [c] Model included vegetables (including 100% juice and potatoes), fruit (including 100% juice), dairy (including flavored milk), SSBs (including flavored milk), whole grains, refined grains, meats, and legumes. [d] Model included vegetables (excluding 100% juice), fruit (excluding 100% juice), dairy (excluding flavored milk), SSBs (excluding flavored milk), whole grains, refined grains, meats, and legumes. [e] Model was the same as the second model, replacing vegetables (excluding 100% juice) with vegetables (excluding 100% juice and potatoes). *A priori* covariates included: age, sex, race/ethnicity, free/reduced lunch status, BMI z-score, day of the week, and total energy.

3.4. Relationships between Breakfast Consumption and Breakfast Dietary Parameters

The relationships between BCG and breakfast dietary parameters are presented in Table 5. INTERMITTENT consumed lower energy at breakfast than REGULAR ($\beta = -207.11$; $p < 0.001$). Consumption of total fiber at breakfast was lower in INTERMITTENT compared to REGULAR ($\beta = -1.75$; $p < 0.001$). Specifically, both soluble and insoluble fiber consumption was lower in INTERMITTENT compared to REGULAR ($\beta = -0.62$ & $\beta = -1.11$, respectively; both $p < 0.001$). Consumption of whole grains at breakfast was lower in INTERMITTENT compared to REGULAR ($\beta = -0.22$; $p < 0.001$).

Table 5. Multivariate regression models of breakfast nutrient intake and breakfast food servings with regular consumers as the referent group ($n = 557$).

Variable	Intermittent		
	β	(95% CI)	p
Breakfast Dietary Intake Parameters			
Breakfast total energy (kcal)	−207.11	(−208.88, −159.76)	<0.001 *
Breakfast protein (%kcal) [a,b]	−0.34	(−1.13, 0.44)	0.13
Breakfast fat (%kcal) [a,b]	0.51	(−1.80, 2.82)	0.59
Breakfast carbohydrate (%kcal) [a,b]	−0.37	(−3.24, 2.51)	0.43
Breakfast total fiber (g) [a]	−1.75	(−2.07, −1.43)	<0.001 *
Breakfast total sugar (%kcal) [a]	−0.61	(−3.12, 1.89)	0.63
Breakfast soluble fiber (g) [b]	−0.62	(−0.74, −0.51)	<0.001 *
Breakfast insoluble fiber (g) [b]	−1.11	(−1.34, −0.87)	<0.001 *
Breakfast added sugar (%kcal) [b]	1.38	(−0.52, 3.29)	0.81
Breakfast Food Servings			
Breakfast whole grains (serving/day) [c]	−0.22	(−0.31, −0.13)	<0.001 *
Breakfast refined grains (serving/day) [c]	−0.03	(−0.12, 0.07)	0.14

* Indicates a statistically significant value of $p < 0.05$. Multivariate regression assessed relationships between all dietary parameters by breakfast consumption groups ($n = 557$). Regular consumers served as the referent group for all analyses. Overall effects not reported due to contrast of only two levels of breakfast consumption groups. Breakfast energy was assessed in a univariate model, adjusting for subsequent energy. [a] Model included breakfast percent protein, percent fat, percent carbohydrate, total fiber, and percent total sugar. [b] Model included breakfast percent protein, percent fat, percent carbohydrate, soluble fiber, insoluble fiber, and percent added sugar. [c] Model included breakfast whole and refined grain servings. A priori covariates included: age, sex, race/ethnicity, free/reduced lunch status, BMI z-score, day of the week, and total energy.

4. Discussion

Contrary to the hypothesis, this study evaluating low-income, Hispanic elementary school-aged children found no protective effects of breakfast consumption on adiposity and metabolic parameters. While regular breakfast consumption was linked to higher daily consumption of total and added sugar, it was also related to higher total HEI-2015 dietary quality scores; higher daily protein, carbohydrate, and fruit juice intake; and lower daily fat and energy intake. Furthermore, regular breakfast consumers had higher energy, fiber, and whole grain consumption in the breakfast meal compared to intermittent breakfast consumers. The link between breakfast consumption and both unhealthy and healthy dietary intake may explain the null effects of breakfast on adiposity and metabolic outcomes.

Similar to the results in this study, other recent studies have shown null or positive associations between breakfast consumption and obesity prevalence [26–30]. Fayet-Moore et al. showed breakfast consumption to be associated with lower overweight and obesity prevalence in children [13]. However, one year later, Fayet-Moore et al. examined breakfast consumption and breakfast cereal choice on anthropometric parameters in a similar cohort and observed no associations between breakfast consumption and overweight and obesity prevalence [28]. A longitudinal study showed increased breakfast consumption to be associated with higher obesity incidence and prevalence following an intervention spanning two and a half years [29]. These findings suggest that quantity and quality of foods consumed at breakfast may play a vital role in contributing to the potential cardiometabolic benefits associated with breakfast consumption.

Comparing breakfast consumption groups, skippers and intermittent breakfast consumers had less eating occasions, on average. However, this was to be expected as these groups are compared to those consistently consuming one main meal of the day. Both skippers and intermittent breakfast consumers had lower HEI-2015 scores than regular breakfast consumers. The USDA reports that children (6–17 years of age) have an average HEI-2015 score of 53 out of 100, which is the lowest of all other age groups [53]. The average HEI-2015 score in the current study was 53.8, similar to the national average for children in this age range [53]. Higher dietary quality was observed in regular consumers, with an HEI-2015 score approximately 3.9 and 2.7 points higher than skippers and intermittent consumers, respectively. These results are consistent with other studies showing that those who consume breakfast have higher diet quality [5,28,30,54,55].

Aside from overall dietary quality, those who regularly consumed breakfast had lower daily intake of fat and higher daily intake of protein, factors that are typically associated with reducing adiposity [56–58]. Though intermittent consumers had a lower number of eating occasions, this group managed to consume approximately 175 kilocalories more than regular breakfast consumers on a daily basis. Breakfast consumption has been associated with higher daily energy [55], but regular breakfast consumers still had lower daily energy intake than intermittent consumers. Regular breakfast consumers had higher daily servings of whole grains than skippers, likely contributing to the higher total and soluble fiber consumption observed. Literature supports that whole grain consumption is associated with decreased adiposity as well [59]. Though regular breakfast consumers had higher daily intake of protein and whole grains and lower daily intake of fat, this group also had higher daily intake of carbohydrates, total sugar, and fruit (including 100% juice) than both breakfast skippers and intermittent consumers. In addition, regular breakfast consumers had higher daily intake of added sugar than breakfast skippers. The relationships between fruit was attenuated when excluding 100% juice, suggesting that breakfast consumption of those beverages was driving the relationships observed with daily carbohydrate and total sugar intake. A similar trend was observed with dairy (including flavored milk), where lower consumption was observed in skippers than regular breakfast consumers. It is well-established that sugar consumption is positively associated with adiposity and blood glucose [60–63] and that whole fruit consumption leads to a greater reduction in hunger than consuming the same amount in fruit juice, with soluble fiber serving a prominent role [64,65]. Flood-Obbagy et al. showed that whole fruit consumption increased satiety more than fruit, fruit juice, and fruit juice with fiber, independent of energy density or fiber content [66]. Despite regular breakfast consumers having higher daily consumption of fruit juice than skippers and intermittent consumers, daily soluble fiber consumption remained superior. These results suggest that replacing fruit juice consumption with whole fruit consumption could further increase dietary quality and, in turn, improve cardiometabolic outcomes. Barr et al. reported higher sugar intake as dietary quality increased in breakfast consumers but suggested this could be due to higher fruit intakes observed [55]. Daily consumption of 100% fruit juice was driving the relationship with fruit in this study while contributing to total and added sugar consumption. Thus, it is possible that higher consumption of fruit juice and added sugar from other dietary sources resulted in deleterious effects of beneficial dietary intake, such as higher protein and whole grain consumption, contributing to the null results of breakfast consumption on anthropometric and metabolic parameters.

Relationships were observed in breakfast dietary parameters between regular and intermittent consumers. Intermittent consumers had lower energy, total fiber, soluble fiber, insoluble fiber, and whole grain consumption at breakfast compared to regular consumers. It is reported that Hispanic children (6–11 years of age) consume approximately 23% of energy at breakfast [67]. This study showed regular breakfast consumers had approximately 184 kilocalories more at breakfast than intermittent breakfast consumers, which is a difference of approximately 10–13% of daily energy for children of this age [68]. Daily energy was higher in intermittent consumers, so this is likely due to consumption of foods at other eating occasions throughout the day. In children, energy intake at breakfast has been shown to be homogenous across tertiles of dietary quality [55]. This compounded with the magnitude of caloric difference observed in the present study highlights the importance of promoting consumption of high-quality breakfast meals. In addition, previous work has shown intakes of carbohydrates and sugars at breakfast to be higher relative to breakfast energy [32]. Relationships between breakfast macronutrient consumption and breakfast sugar consumption were not observed between regular and intermittent consumers, however. While intermittent breakfast consumption was linked to lower soluble fiber intake at breakfast than regular breakfast consumption, the difference is relatively small at 0.62 g. Lower total fiber, soluble fiber, and insoluble fiber intake at breakfast was observed in intermittent consumers compared to regular consumers. Of the 1.75 g lower of total fiber, majority was insoluble fiber, which contributed 1.11 g. It can be postulated that the lower whole grain intake of 0.22 servings at breakfast observed in intermittent consumers contributed to these fiber results. However, the differences in fiber and whole grain content at breakfast were relatively small and lend little interpretation. The results observed propose dietary patterns surrounding breakfast consumption in this population may only differ primarily in energy content.

While both breakfast skippers and intermittent consumers had lower daily sugar intake than regular consumers, only breakfast skippers had lower daily added sugar intake than regular consumers. Added sugar was represented as percent of daily energy in this study. The insignificance of daily added sugar between intermittent and regular consumers highlights that, regardless of the higher daily energy observed, intermittent consumers had a similar percentage of added sugar intake to that of regular consumers. Sugar consumption has been studied as a food addiction [69]. Looking at food addiction in children with overweight, Filgueiras et al. showed that 95% of children (n = 139) showed at least one sign of food addiction, with 24% being diagnosed with food addiction and higher added sugar and ultra-processed food consumption as main contributors to food addiction [70]. The present study showed that breakfast consumers had higher daily consumption of total sugars, added sugars, and carbohydrates. These nutrients have properties of addiction, and consumption of breakfast meals composed of higher added sugar has been associated with higher added sugar consumption throughout the day [71]. As a result, this study posits a possible rationale for null relationships observed between breakfast consumption and cardiometabolic outcomes, suggesting that breakfast quality should be addressed in future interventions and guidelines.

Limitations and Strengths

The current study had some limitations for consideration. First, the study was cross-sectional, thus causality cannot be inferred. This data, however, was baseline data from a randomized controlled trial. Therefore, future analyses will examine interventional effects of breakfast consumption on cardiometabolic outcomes and dietary intake in this population. The sample is predominantly Hispanic, so we were unable to distinguish any breakfast patterns or dietary composition by race or ethnicity. In addition, nearly 49% of children in this sample are classified as having overweight or obesity, so the sample is rather homogenous, and breakfast may not have a robust effect to elicit a response in our population. However, given the higher prevalence rates of obesity in Hispanic youth [1], it is important to examine dietary behaviors that are linked to obesity in this high-risk homogenous population. Another limitation to the current study is that there is no standard definition of breakfast, especially in the context of children, so it is possible that some of these results could be due to the chosen definition. The *Dietary Guidelines for Americans, 2015–2020* does not contain a standardized definition or recommendation for breakfast [68]. The energy cut point of 15% daily energy was chosen to exclude meals that were very low or no energy foods and beverages, i.e., a glass of water, single banana, nutrition bar, etc. Furthermore, the recommended amount of energy to be consumed at breakfast is dependent on the total number of EOs throughout the day [47]. Due to the lower number of EOs observed in Hispanic children (6–11 years of age) from the *What We Eat in America* data tables, the lower end of 15% daily energy proved appropriate for the breakfast definition in this study and has been recommended as the minimum energy requirement [47,72]. The recommendation for the breakfast energy threshold is 25%, but Hispanic children (6–11 years of age) consume, on average, 23% of daily energy at breakfast, so an upper limit of 25% did not seem appropriate [47,67].

One notable strength of the study is that dietary recalls were collected for two days, permitting the use of a definitive measure of dietary intake and evaluation of breakfast composition while controlling for confounding dietary variables. In turn, this study was able to discern and examine three breakfast consumption patterns (skipper, intermittent, and regular) instead of only two (eaters and skippers) seen in other studies. Dietary recall methodology allowed this study to examine different patterns of breakfast consumption on breakfast composition. One limitation, however, is that two dietary recalls may not be indicative of regular dietary behaviors.

5. Conclusions

Breakfast consumption was not associated with lower adiposity or healthier metabolic parameters, but regular breakfast consumption was linked to higher total HEI-2015 dietary quality scores; higher daily consumption of protein, carbohydrates, fruit juice, and whole grains; lower daily consumption of energy and dietary fat; and higher consumption of energy, fiber, and whole grains at breakfast. However, this study proposes that higher sugar intake of breakfast consumers played a role in masking the relationship with breakfast on adiposity and metabolic parameters. The results suggest that quality of foods consumed at breakfast plays a pivotal role in whether or not benefits of breakfast consumption are received.

Author Contributions: Conceptualization, J.N.D., H.J.L., and M.R.J.; methodology, J.N.D., H.J.L., and M.R.J.; software, M.R.J.; validation, J.N.D. and M.R.J.; formal analysis, J.N.D., H.J.L., and M.R.J.; investigation, J.N.D., H.J.L., M.R.J., F.M.A., M.J.L., S.V., and R.G.; resources, J.N.D., H.J.L., and M.R.J.; data curation, J.N.D. and M.R.J.; writing—original draft preparation, J.N.D., H.J.L., and M.R.J.; writing—review and editing, J.N.D., H.J.L., M.R.J., F.M.A., M.J.L., S.V., and R.G.; visualization, J.N.D., H.J.L., M.R.J.; supervision, J.N.D. and H.J.L.; project administration, J.N.D.; funding acquisition, J.N.D. All authors have read and agreed to the published version of the manuscript.

Funding: This research was funded by the National Institutes of Health, National Heart, Lung, and Blood Institute, Grant No. R01HL123865.

Acknowledgments: The authors thank all of the students and their families for participating in this study and extend great appreciation to the TX Sprouts staff for their monumental contributions to the intervention and all collected measurements.

Conflicts of Interest: The authors declare no conflicts of interest.

References

1. Hales, C.M.; Carroll, M.D.; Fryar, C.D.; Ogden, C.L. Prevalence of obesity among adults and youth: United States, 2015–2016. *NCHS Data Brief.* **2017**, *288*, 1–8.
2. Monzani, A.; Ricotti, R.; Caputo, M.; Solito, A.; Archero, F.; Bellone, S.; Prodam, F. A systematic review of the association of skipping breakfast with weight and cardiometabolic risk factors in children and adolescents. What should we better investigate in the future? *Nutrients* **2019**, *11*, 387. [CrossRef] [PubMed]
3. Smith, K.J.; Gall, S.L.; McNaughton, S.A.; Blizzard, L.; Dwyer, T.; Venn, A.J. Skipping breakfast: Longitudinal associations with cardiometabolic risk factors in the Childhood determinants of adult health study. *Am. J. Clin. Nutr.* **2010**, *92*, 1316–1325. [CrossRef] [PubMed]
4. Shafiee, G.; Kelishadi, R.; Qorbani, M.; Motlagh, M.E.; Taheri, M.; Ardalan, G.; Taslimi, M.; Poursafa, P.; Heshmat, R.; Larijani, B. Association of breakfast intake with cardiometabolic risk factors. *J. Pediatr.* **2013**, *89*, 575–582. [CrossRef] [PubMed]
5. Ho, C.Y.; Huang, Y.C.; Lo, Y.T.; Wahlqvist, M.L.; Lee, M.S. Breakfast is associated with the metabolic syndrome and school performance among Taiwanese children. *Res. Dev. Disabil.* **2015**, *43–44*, 179–188. [CrossRef]

6. Bauer, L.B.; Reynolds, L.J.; Douglas, S.M.; Kearney, M.L.; Hoertel, H.A.; Shafer, R.S.; Thyfault, J.P.; Leidy, H.J. A pilot study examining the effects of consuming a high-protein vs normal-protein breakfast on free-living glycemic control in overweight/obese 'breakfast skipping' adolescents. *Int. J. Obes.* **2015**, *39*, 1421–1424. [CrossRef] [PubMed]
7. Deshmukh-Taskar, P.; Nicklas, T.A.; Radcliffe, J.D.; O'Neil, C.E.; Liu, Y. The relationship of breakfast skipping and type of breakfast consumed with overweight/obesity, abdominal obesity, other cardiometabolic risk factors and the metabolic syndrome in young adults. The National Health and Nutrition Examination Survey (NHANES): 1999–2006. *Public Health Nutr.* **2013**, *16*, 2073–2082. [CrossRef]
8. Monzani, A.; Rapa, A.; Fuiano, N.; Diddi, G.; Prodam, F.; Bellone, S.; Bona, G. Metabolic syndrome is strictly associated with parental obesity beginning from childhood. *Clin. Endocrinol.* **2014**, *81*, 45–51. [CrossRef]
9. Osawa, H.; Sugihara, N.; Ukiya, T.; Ishizuka, Y.; Birkhed, D.; Hasegawa, M.; Matsukubo, T. Metabolic syndrome, lifestyle, and dental caries in Japanese school children. *Bull. Tokyo Dent. Coll.* **2015**, *56*, 233–241. [CrossRef]
10. O'Neil, C.E.; Nicklas, T.A.; Fulgoni, V.L., 3rd. Nutrient intake, diet quality, and weight measures in breakfast patterns consumed by children compared with breakfast skippers: NHANES 2001–2008. *AIMS Public Health* **2015**, *2*, 441–468. [CrossRef]
11. Smetanina, N.; Albaviciute, E.; Babinska, V.; Karinauskiene, L.; Albertsson-Wikland, K.; Petrauskiene, A.; Verkauskiene, R. Prevalence of overweight/obesity in relation to dietary habits and lifestyle among 7–17 years old children and adolescents in Lithuania. *BMC Public Health* **2015**, *15*, 1001. [CrossRef] [PubMed]
12. Zakrzewski, J.K.; Gillison, F.B.; Cumming, S.; Church, T.S.; Katzmarzyk, P.T.; Broyles, S.T.; Champagne, C.M.; Chaput, J.P.; Denstel, K.D.; Fogelholm, M.; et al. Associations between breakfast frequency and adiposity indicators in children from 12 countries. *Int. J. Obes. Suppl.* **2015**, *5*, S80–S88. [CrossRef] [PubMed]
13. Fayet-Moore, F.; Kim, J.; Sritharan, N.; Petocz, P. Impact of breakfast skipping and breakfast choice on the nutrient intake and body mass index of australian children. *Nutrients* **2016**, *8*, 487. [CrossRef] [PubMed]
14. Smith, K.J.; Breslin, M.C.; McNaughton, S.A.; Gall, S.L.; Blizzard, L.; Venn, A.J. Skipping breakfast among Australian children and adolescents; findings from the 2011–12 national nutrition and physical activity survey. *Aust. N. Z. J. Public Health* **2017**, *41*, 572–578. [CrossRef] [PubMed]
15. Gotthelf, S.J.; Tempestti, C.P. Breakfast, nutritional status, and socioeconomic outcome measures among primary school students from the City of Salta: A cross-sectional study. *Arch. Argent. Pediatr.* **2017**, *115*, 424–431. [CrossRef]
16. Nilsen, B.B.; Yngve, A.; Monteagudo, C.; Tellstrom, R.; Scander, H.; Werner, B. Reported habitual intake of breakfast and selected foods in relation to overweight status among seven- to nine-year-old Swedish children. *Scand. J. Public Health* **2017**, *45*, 886–894. [CrossRef]
17. Tee, E.S.; Nurliyana, A.R.; Norimah, A.K.; Mohamed, H.; Tan, S.Y.; Appukutty, M.; Hopkins, S.; Thielecke, F.; Ong, M.K.; Ning, C.; et al. Breakfast consumption among Malaysian primary and secondary school children and relationship with body weight status—Findings from the MyBreakfast Study. *Asia Pac. J. Clin. Nutr.* **2018**, *27*, 421–432. [CrossRef]
18. Archero, F.; Ricotti, R.; Solito, A.; Carrera, D.; Civello, F.; Di Bella, R.; Bellone, S.; Prodam, F. Adherence to the mediterranean diet among school children and adolescents living in northern italy and unhealthy food behaviors associated to overweight. *Nutrients* **2018**, *10*, 1322. [CrossRef]
19. Gibney, M.J.; Barr, S.I.; Bellisle, F.; Drewnowski, A.; Fagt, S.; Livingstone, B.; Masset, G.; Varela Moreiras, G.; Moreno, L.A.; Smith, J.; et al. Breakfast in human nutrition: The international breakfast research initiative. *Nutrients* **2018**, *10*, 559. [CrossRef]
20. Currie, C.Z.C.; Morgan, A.; Currie, D.; de Looze, M.; Roberts, C.; Samdal, O.; Smith, O.R.F.; Barnekow, V. (Eds.) Social determinants of health and well-being among young people. In *Health Behaviour in School-Aged Children (HBSC) Study: International Report from the 2009/2010 Survey*; World Health Organization: Copenhagen, Denmark, 2012; p. 252.
21. Murata, M. Secular trends in growth and changes in eating patterns of Japanese children. *Am. J. Clin. Nutr.* **2000**, *72*, 1379S–1383S. [CrossRef]
22. Dwyer, J.T.; Evans, M.; Stone, E.J.; Feldman, H.A.; Lytle, L.; Hoelscher, D.; Johnson, C.; Zive, M.; Yang, M. Child and adolescents' eating patterns influence their nutrient intakes. *J. Am. Diet. Assoc.* **2001**, *101*, 798–802. [CrossRef]

23. Van Kleef, E.; Vingerhoeds, M.H.; Vrijhof, M.; van Trijp, H.C.M. Breakfast barriers and opportunities for children living in a Dutch disadvantaged neighbourhood. *Appetite* **2016**, *107*, 372–382. [CrossRef] [PubMed]
24. Papas, M.A.; Trabulsi, J.C.; Dahl, A.; Dominick, G. Food insecurity increases the odds of obesity among young hispanic children. *J. Immigr. Minor. Health* **2016**, *18*, 1046–1052. [CrossRef] [PubMed]
25. Potochnick, S.; Perreira, K.M.; Bravin, J.I.; Castaneda, S.F.; Daviglus, M.L.; Gallo, L.C.; Isasi, C.R. Food insecurity among hispanic/latino youth: Who is at risk and what are the health correlates? *J. Adolesc. Health* **2019**, *64*, 631–639. [CrossRef] [PubMed]
26. Kuriyan, R.; Thomas, T.; Sumithra, S.; Lokesh, D.P.; Sheth, N.R.; Joy, R.; Bhat, S.; Kurpad, A.V. Potential factors related to waist circumference in urban South Indian children. *Indian Pediatr.* **2012**, *49*, 124–128. [CrossRef]
27. Kupers, L.K.; de Pijper, J.J.; Sauer, P.J.; Stolk, R.P.; Corpeleijn, E. Skipping breakfast and overweight in 2- and 5-year-old Dutch children-the GECKO Drenthe cohort. *Int. J. Obes.* **2014**, *38*, 569–571. [CrossRef]
28. Fayet-Moore, F.; McConnell, A.; Tuck, K.; Petocz, P. Breakfast and breakfast cereal choice and its impact on nutrient and sugar intakes and anthropometric measures among a nationally representative sample of australian children and adolescents. *Nutrients* **2017**, *9*, 1045. [CrossRef]
29. Polonsky, H.M.; Bauer, K.W.; Fisher, J.O.; Davey, A.; Sherman, S.; Abel, M.L.; Hanlon, A.; Ruth, K.J.; Dale, L.C.; Foster, G.D. Effect of a breakfast in the classroom initiative on obesity in urban school-aged children: A cluster randomized clinical trial. *JAMA Pediatr.* **2019**, *173*, 326–333. [CrossRef]
30. Coulthard, J.D.; Palla, L.; Pot, G.K. Breakfast consumption and nutrient intakes in 4–18-year-olds: UK national diet and nutrition survey rolling programme (2008–2012). *Br. J. Nutr.* **2017**, *118*, 280–290. [CrossRef]
31. Deshmukh-Taskar, P.R.; Nicklas, T.A.; O'Neil, C.E.; Keast, D.R.; Radcliffe, J.D.; Cho, S. The relationship of breakfast skipping and type of breakfast consumption with nutrient intake and weight status in children and adolescents: The National health and nutrition examination survey 1999–2006. *J. Am. Diet. Assoc.* **2010**, *110*, 869–878. [CrossRef]
32. Drewnowski, A.; Rehm, C.D.; Vieux, F. Breakfast in the United States: Food and nutrient intakes in relation to diet quality in national health and examination survey 2011–2014. a study from the international breakfast research initiative. *Nutrients* **2018**, *10*, 1200. [CrossRef] [PubMed]
33. Lepicard, E.M.; Maillot, M.; Vieux, F.; Viltard, M.; Bonnet, F. Quantitative and qualitative analysis of breakfast nutritional composition in French schoolchildren aged 9–11 years. *J. Hum. Nutr. Diet.* **2017**, *30*, 151–158. [CrossRef] [PubMed]
34. Davis, J.; Nikah, K.; Asigbee, F.M.; Landry, M.J.; Vandyousefi, S.; Ghaddar, R.; Hoover, A.; Jeans, M.; Pont, S.J.; Richards, D.; et al. Design and participant characteristics of TX sprouts: A school-based cluster randomized gardening, nutrition, and cooking intervention. *Contemp Clin. Trials* **2019**, *85*, 105834. [CrossRef] [PubMed]
35. Centers for Disease Control and Prevention. Anthropometry Procedures Manual. 2007. Available online: https://www.cdc.gov/nchs/data/nhanes/nhanes_07_08/manual_an.pdf (accessed on 7 July 2020).
36. Centers for Disease Control and Prevention. Clinical Growth Charts. 2000. Available online: https://www.cdc.gov/growthcharts/clinical_charts.htm (accessed on 7 July 2020).
37. American Diabetes, A. Diagnosis and classification of diabetes mellitus. *Diabetes Care* **2014**, *37* (Suppl. 1), S81–S90. [CrossRef]
38. Friedewald, W.T.; Levy, R.I.; Fredrickson, D.S. Estimation of the concentration of low-density lipoprotein cholesterol in plasma, without use of the preparative ultracentrifuge. *Clin. Chem.* **1972**, *18*, 499–502. [CrossRef]
39. Burrows, T.L.; Martin, R.J.; Collins, C.E. A systematic review of the validity of dietary assessment methods in children when compared with the method of doubly labeled water. *J. Am. Diet. Assoc.* **2010**, *110*, 1501–1510. [CrossRef]
40. Feskanich, D.; Sielaff, B.H.; Chong, K.; Buzzard, I.M. Computerized collection and analysis of dietary intake information. *Comput. Methods Programs Biomed.* **1989**, *30*, 47–57. [CrossRef]
41. National Cancer Institute. Developing the Healthy Eating Index. 2015. Available online: https://epi.grants.cancer.gov/hei/developing.html (accessed on 7 July 2020).
42. Kirkpatrick, S.I.; Reedy, J.; Krebs-Smith, S.M.; Pannucci, T.E.; Subar, A.F.; Wilson, M.M.; Lerman, J.L.; Tooze, J.A. Applications of the healthy eating index for surveillance, epidemiology, and intervention research: Considerations and caveats. *J. Acad. Nutr. Diet.* **2018**, *118*, 1603–1621. [CrossRef]

43. Krebs-Smith, S.M.; Pannucci, T.E.; Subar, A.F.; Kirkpatrick, S.I.; Lerman, J.L.; Tooze, J.A.; Wilson, M.M.; Reedy, J. Update of the healthy eating index: HEI-2015. *J. Acad. Nutr. Diet.* **2018**, *118*, 1591–1602. [CrossRef]
44. Reedy, J.; Lerman, J.L.; Krebs-Smith, S.M.; Kirkpatrick, S.I.; Pannucci, T.E.; Wilson, M.M.; Subar, A.F.; Kahle, L.L.; Tooze, J.A. Evaluation of the healthy eating index-2015. *J. Acad. Nutr. Diet.* **2018**, *118*, 1622–1633. [CrossRef]
45. Johnson, R.K.; Driscoll, P.; Goran, M.I. Comparison of multiple-pass 24-hour recall estimates of energy intake with total energy expenditure determined by the doubly labeled water method in young children. *J. Am. Diet. Assoc.* **1996**, *96*, 1140–1144. [CrossRef]
46. Leech, R.M.; Worsley, A.; Timperio, A.; McNaughton, S.A. Characterizing eating patterns: A comparison of eating occasion definitions. *Am. J. Clin. Nutr.* **2015**, *102*, 1229–1237. [CrossRef] [PubMed]
47. O'Neil, C.E.; Byrd-Bredbenner, C.; Hayes, D.; Jana, L.; Klinger, S.E.; Stephenson-Martin, S. The role of breakfast in health: Definition and criteria for a quality breakfast. *J. Acad. Nutr. Diet.* **2014**, *114*, S8–S26. [CrossRef] [PubMed]
48. Pereira, M.A.; Erickson, E.; McKee, P.; Schrankler, K.; Raatz, S.K.; Lytle, L.A.; Pellegrini, A.D. Breakfast frequency and quality may affect glycemia and appetite in adults and children. *J. Nutr.* **2011**, *141*, 163–168. [CrossRef] [PubMed]
49. Siega-Riz, A.M.; Popkin, B.M.; Carson, T. Trends in breakfast consumption for children in the United States from 1965–1991. *Am. J. Clin. Nutr.* **1998**, *67*, 748S–756S. [CrossRef]
50. Cho, S.; Dietrich, M.; Brown, C.J.; Clark, C.A.; Block, G. The effect of breakfast type on total daily energy intake and body mass index: Results from the third national health and nutrition examination survey (NHANES III). *J. Am. Coll. Nutr.* **2003**, *22*, 296–302. [CrossRef]
51. Deshmukh-Taskar, P.R.; Radcliffe, J.D.; Liu, Y.; Nicklas, T.A. Do breakfast skipping and breakfast type affect energy intake, nutrient intake, nutrient adequacy, and diet quality in young adults? NHANES 1999–2002. *J. Am. Coll. Nutr.* **2010**, *29*, 407–418. [CrossRef]
52. Lyerly, J.E.; Huber, L.R.; Warren-Findlow, J.; Racine, E.F.; Dmochowski, J. Is breakfast skipping associated with physical activity among U.S. adolescents? A cross-sectional study of adolescents aged 12–19 years, National Health and Nutrition Examination Survey (NHANES). *Public Health Nutr.* **2014**, *17*, 896–905. [CrossRef]
53. United States Department of Agriculture. HEI Scores for Americans. Average Healthy Eating Index-2015 Scores for Americans by Age Group, WWEIA/NHANES 2015–2016. 2016. Available online: https://fns-azureedge.net/sites/default/files/media/file/HEI-2015_1516_web.pdf (accessed on 7 July 2020).
54. Gaal, S.; Kerr, M.A.; Ward, M.; McNulty, H.; Livingstone, M.B.E. Breakfast consumption in the UK: Patterns, nutrient intake and diet quality. A study from the international breakfast research initiative group. *Nutrients* **2018**, *10*, 999. [CrossRef]
55. Barr, S.I.; Vatanparast, H.; Smith, J. Breakfast in Canada: Prevalence of consumption, contribution to nutrient and food group intakes, and variability across tertiles of daily diet quality. A study from the international breakfast research initiative. *Nutrients* **2018**, *10*, 985. [CrossRef]
56. Chaumontet, C.; Even, P.C.; Schwarz, J.; Simonin-Foucault, A.; Piedcoq, J.; Fromentin, G.; Azzout-Marniche, D.; Tome, D. High dietary protein decreases fat deposition induced by high-fat and high-sucrose diet in rats. *Br. J. Nutr.* **2015**, *114*, 1132–1142. [CrossRef] [PubMed]
57. French, W.W.; Dridi, S.; Shouse, S.A.; Wu, H.; Hawley, A.; Lee, S.O.; Gu, X.; Baum, J.I. A High-protein diet reduces weight gain, decreases food intake, decreases liver fat deposition, and improves markers of muscle metabolism in obese zucker Rats. *Nutrients* **2017**, *9*, 587. [CrossRef] [PubMed]
58. Wang, L.; Du, S.; Wang, H.; Popkin, B. Influence of dietary fat intake on bodyweight and risk of obesity among Chinese adults, 1991–2015: A prospective cohort study. *Lancet* **2018**, *392*. [CrossRef]
59. Harland, J.I.; Garton, L.E. Whole-grain intake as a marker of healthy body weight and adiposity. *Public Health Nutr.* **2008**, *11*, 554–563. [CrossRef] [PubMed]
60. Wang, J.; Shang, L.; Light, K.; O'Loughlin, J.; Paradis, G.; Gray-Donald, K. Associations between added sugar (solid vs. liquid) intakes, diet quality, and adiposity indicators in Canadian children. *Appl. Physiol. Nutr. Metab.* **2015**, *40*, 835–841. [CrossRef] [PubMed]
61. Bigornia, S.J.; LaValley, M.P.; Noel, S.E.; Moore, L.L.; Ness, A.R.; Newby, P.K. Sugar-sweetened beverage consumption and central and total adiposity in older children: A prospective study accounting for dietary reporting errors. *Public Health Nutr.* **2015**, *18*, 1155–1163. [CrossRef] [PubMed]

62. Laverty, A.A.; Magee, L.; Monteiro, C.A.; Saxena, S.; Millett, C. Sugar and artificially sweetened beverage consumption and adiposity changes: National longitudinal study. *Int. J. Behav. Nutr. Phys. Act.* **2015**, *12*, 137. [CrossRef]
63. Seferidi, P.; Millett, C.; Laverty, A.A. Sweetened beverage intake in association to energy and sugar consumption and cardiometabolic markers in children. *Pediatr. Obes.* **2018**, *13*, 195–203. [CrossRef]
64. Mattes, R. Soup and satiety. *Physiol. Behav.* **2005**, *83*, 739–747. [CrossRef]
65. Bolton, R.P.; Heaton, K.W.; Burroughs, L.F. The role of dietary fiber in satiety, glucose, and insulin: Studies with fruit and fruit juice. *Am. J. Clin. Nutr.* **1981**, *34*, 211–217. [CrossRef]
66. Flood-Obbagy, J.E.; Rolls, B.J. The effect of fruit in different forms on energy intake and satiety at a meal. *Appetite* **2009**, *52*, 416–422. [CrossRef] [PubMed]
67. US Department of Agriculture. Percentages of Selected Nutrients Contributed by Food and Beverages Consumed at Breakfast, by Race/Ethnicity and Age. What We Eat. In America NHANES 2015–2016. Available online: https://www.ars.usda.gov/ARSUserFiles/80400530/pdf/1516/Table_14_BRK_RAC_15.pdf (accessed on 7 July 2020).
68. US. Department of Health and Human Services; U.S. Department of Agriculture. *Dietary Guidelines for Americans, 2015–2020*, 8th ed.; U.S. Government Printing Office: Washington, DC, USA, 2015.
69. Lennerz, B.; Lennerz, J.K. Food Addiction, High-Glycemic-Index Carbohydrates, and Obesity. *Clin. Chem.* **2018**, *64*, 64–71. [CrossRef] [PubMed]
70. Filgueiras, A.R.; Pires de Almeida, V.B.; Koch Nogueira, P.C.; Alvares Domene, S.M.; Eduardo da Silva, C.; Sesso, R.; Sawaya, A.L. Exploring the consumption of ultra-processed foods and its association with food addiction in overweight children. *Appetite* **2019**, *135*, 137–145. [CrossRef]
71. Afeiche, M.C.; Taillie, L.S.; Hopkins, S.; Eldridge, A.L.; Popkin, B.M. Breakfast dietary patterns among mexican children are related to total-day diet quality. *J. Nutr.* **2017**, *147*, 404–412. [CrossRef] [PubMed]
72. US Department of Agriculture, A.R.S. Distribution of Meal Patterns and Snack Occasions, by Race/Ethnicity and Age. What We Eat. In America NHANES 2015–2016. Available online: https://www.ars.usda.gov/ARSUserFiles/80400530/pdf/1516/Table_34_DMP_RAC_15.pdf (accessed on 8 July 2020).

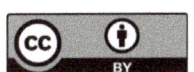 © 2020 by the authors. Licensee MDPI, Basel, Switzerland. This article is an open access article distributed under the terms and conditions of the Creative Commons Attribution (CC BY) license (http://creativecommons.org/licenses/by/4.0/).

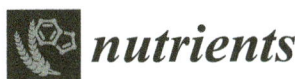

Article

Food Involvement, Eating Restrictions and Dietary Patterns in Polish Adults: Expected Effects of Their Relationships (LifeStyle Study)

Marzena Jezewska-Zychowicz, Jerzy Gębski * and Milena Kobylińska

Institute of Human Nutrition Sciences, Warsaw University of Life Sciences (SGGW-WULS), Nowoursynowska 159C, 02-776 Warsaw, Poland; marzena_jezewska_zychowicz@sggw.pl (M.J.-Z.); milena_wasilewska@wp.pl (M.K.)
* Correspondence: jerzy_gebski@sggw.pl; Tel.: +48-22-593-7137

Received: 26 March 2020; Accepted: 21 April 2020; Published: 24 April 2020

Abstract: Understanding the factors that coexist with healthy and unhealthy eating behaviors is prevalent and important for public health. The aim of this study was to investigate the associations between food involvement, eating restrictions, and dietary patterns in a representative sample of Polish adults. The study was conducted among a group of 1007 adults. Questions with the answers yes or no were used to obtain the data regarding eating restrictions. Data relating to food involvement were obtained with the Food Involvement Scale (FIS). Questions from the Beliefs and Eating Habits questionnaire were used to measure the frequency of consumption of different food groups. Five dietary patterns (DPs) were derived using principal component analysis (PCA), i.e., 'Fruit and vegetables', 'Wholemeal food', 'Fast foods and sweets', 'Fruit and vegetable juices' and "Meat and meat products'. In each of the DPs, three groups of participants were identified based on tertile distribution with the upper tertile denoting the most frequent consumption. Nearly two-thirds of the study sample declared some restrictions in food consumption. The probability of implementing restrictions in consumption of foods high in sugar, fat and high-fat foods increased in the upper tertile of 'Fruit and vegetables' and 'Wholemeal' DPs. Moreover, the probability of implementing restrictions in consumption of meat and high-starch products increased in 'Wholemeal' DP. The probability of using eating restrictions decreased in the upper tertile of 'Fast foods and sweets' and Meat and meat products' DPs. In conclusion, individuals characterized by high food involvement were more inclined to use eating restrictions than individuals with lower food involvement. Their DPs were also healthier compared to those of individuals manifesting low food involvement. Therefore, promoting personal commitment to learning about and experiencing food may be an effective way of inducing a change of eating habits, and therefore a healthier diet.

Keywords: dietary patterns; eating restrictions; food involvement; adults; obesity

1. Introduction

Research indicates that a significant proportion of the population, particularly young women, use various dietary restrictions [1–3]. This practice may have both positive and negative effects on nutritional status, health, and finally on the quality of life. Eating restrictions may lead to unhealthy dietary habits and eating disorders [4]. On the other hand, present-day diets with a high content of fat, sweet, and energy density often correlate with higher body mass index (BMI) [5–7]. Beyond overweight or obesity, such diets can lead to the development of other diet-related chronic diseases, including type 2 diabetes, cardiovascular diseases and some cancers [8]. Therefore, some restraint in consumption of foods, and especially those undesirable in a healthy diet might be beneficial and healthy behavior. For example, calorie restriction provides many benefits for quality of life, especially with respect to loss of weight and fat mass [9,10].

One of the reasons for excessive food consumption and inefficiency in reducing food consumption may be the individuals' interest in food, i.e., food involvement. According to Bell and Marshall [11] food involvement concerns the extent to which a person cares about and is interested in food. The importance of food in a person's life varies across individuals, for example, due to socio-demographic characteristics [12]. Differences are also observed in dietary behaviors. Previous studies have shown that consumers who are more food involved are more sensitive to the sensory properties of food [11]. Highly food-involved individuals may be more inclined towards having new food experiences, i.e., food neophilic [13]. Moreover, individuals with higher involvement tend to make healthier food choices [14,15] but they also may reveal both healthier and less healthy dietary practices [16]. It is still unknown whether this relationship stems from being food-involved or whether healthier choices lead to higher food involvement.

So far, different approaches have been used to measure the construct of food involvement, including but not limited to: a theoretical model of involvement based on expectancy-value theory [17], a large multi-item food-related lifestyle measure [18] or a general involvement measure with the food-provisioning process, the Food Involvement Scale (FIS) [11]. The scale includes preparation, cooking and disposal whichs reflected in the consumers' engagement with food and their experiences, knowledge, skills and competencies [11]. Thus, the FIS can be considered as a general involvement measure rather than a measure of involvement with a specific food item or brand. For this reason, it appears to be useful in explaining the use of restrictions in food consumption, but also food choices that are revealed in dietary patterns [19–21]. The analysis of dietary patterns seems to be a useful approach to explain to what extent healthy choices depend on being more food involved, and also on having greater control over food by using restrictions [22].

Studies have shown that dietary patterns are significantly associated with many disease outcomes or biomarkers, including cardiovascular disease, overweight and obesity, and other diseases [23]. So far, few results have been reported on the association between eating restrictions and dietary patterns [24].

We assumed that individuals who are highly involved with food would be less able to use eating restrictions compared to individuals with lower food involvement. For this reason, it seemed more likely that the dietary patterns of more food-involved people will be less healthy. Therefore, the aim of this study was to investigate the associations between eating restrictions, food involvement, and dietary patterns in a representative sample of Polish adults.

2. Materials and Methods

2.1. Data Collection

Analyses were carried out on data from the LifeStyle Project. A computer-assisted personal interviewing (CAPI) technique was used in a cross-sectional study. Participants were selected from the panel of the research agency ARC Market and Opinion that consists of approximately 55,000 registered individuals. People are invited to the panel both via off-line and online invitations (65% and 35%, respectively).

After being sent an invitation to participate in the survey, 6910 people expressed their willingness to participate in the study. Quota selection regarding gender, age, place of residence and region was used to ensure the representativeness of the Polish population. During the recruitment for the study 5 people did not meet the panel criteria, i.e., adults aged 25–65, 144 people stopped filling out the questionnaire before it was completed, 5746 people did not qualify to the quota. During the collection control stage eight people were removed from the database due to very short time of completing the questionnaire and the lack of differences in answers to all frequency questions (Supplementary Materials Figure S1). The study involved 1007 participants.

2.2. Ethical Approval

The Ethics Committee of the Faculty of Human Nutrition and Consumer Science, Warsaw University of Life Sciences (SGGW) appointed on the basis of Regulation No. 27 of the SGGW Rector of 5 May 2016 approved the protocol of LifeStyle Study on 27 June 2016, Resolution No. 01/2016 as consistent with the guidelines laid down in the Declaration of Helsinki. Informed consent was provided by participants.

2.3. Eating Restrictions

Standardized one-to-one interview (answers yes/no) at respondent's home was used to obtain data regarding eating restrictions. Questions referred to 10 categories of restrictions, while the analyses included only 6 categories which were indicated by at least 5% of study sample, i.e., restrictions in: food quantity, sugar and/or sweets, high-fat foods, fats, cereals and/or bread and/or potatoes, and meats. Other restrictions concerned: fish, dairy products, raw vegetables and raw fruit.

2.4. Dietary Patterns

Questions from Dietary Habits and Nutrition Beliefs Questionnaire–KomPAN [25] were used to measure the frequency of consumption of different food groups, including: wholemeal bread; wholemeal pasta and groats; fermented milk drinks; cheeses (including melted cheese, blue cheese); cured meats and sausages; red meat; white meat; fried foods; fruits; vegetables; vegetable juices; fruit juices; fizzy drinks; meals or snacks such as burgers, pizza, chicken, fries; sweets and cakes; crisps and other salty snacks. To assess the habitual consumption over the past year the question 'How often do you eat . . . .? was used for each food group. Food frequency consumption was evaluated in 6 categories: 'never' (1), 1–3 times a month (2), once a week (3), few times a week (4), once a day (5), and 'few times a day' (6). KomPAN is the questionnaire developed by Polish researchers to evaluate dietary habits, lifestyle and nutrition knowledge whose test-retest reproducibility was assessed among people from all over the country, in healthy subjects and those suffering from chronic diseases [26].

A data-driven (a posteriori) approach was used to identify dietary patterns [23]. PDs were derived by principal component analysis (PCA) to which variables describing frequency of eating some foods were introduced. The factorability of data was confirmed with a Kaiser–Meyer–Olkin (KMO) measure of sampling adequacy and Bartlett's test of sphericity which achieved statistical significance [27]. KMO value was 0.781 which indicates the correct choice of analysis and the number of factors. Bartlett's test had a significance of $p < 0.0001$. To derive dietary patterns a varimax normalized rotation was used in order to extract not correlated factors and obtain high variance explained [27]. Eigenvalues of at least 1.00 were considered. Five dietary patterns were derived: 'Fruit and vegetables', 'Wholemeal food', 'Fast foods and sweets', 'Fruit and vegetable juices' and 'Meat and meat products'. Total variance explained was 64.2%. The relationship between the so-identified dietary patterns and selected elements of the lifestyle was already presented in other articles [28,29].

2.5. Food Involvement

Data relative to food involvement were obtained with the Food Involvement Scale developed in 2002 by Bell and Marshal [11]. The original scale includes 12 items with a Likert scale ranging from (1) "completely disagree" to (7) "completely agree". In this study, the interval between the possible answers was reduced from 7 to 5 points (1—disagree; 2—rather disagree; 3—neither agree nor disagree; 4—rather agree; 5—agree). The original version was translated to Polish and then the instrument was back-translated from Polish to English. Negative statements from original scale were changed to positive statements (without "no"). The Food Involvement score was calculated by the sum of the individual's answers. The higher the score, the greater was the food involvement of the person. The scores obtained ranged from 13 to 60 points.

2.6. Sociodemographic Variables

Considered sociodemographic variables were as follows: gender, age, education, place of residence. Body mass index (BMI) was calculated using self-reported weight and height and categorized according to International Obesity Task Force (IOTF) standards [30].

2.7. Statistical Analysis

Participants in each of the dietary patterns were divided into three groups based on tertile distribution: 1st tertile (T1), 2nd tertile (T2) and 3rd tertile (T3). T3 had the strongest adherence to the pattern while T1 had the weakest one. Median was used to categorize the sample in accordance to food involvement. Scores on the Food Involvement Scale higher than 40 points indicate high food involvement.

Associations between eating restrictions, food involvement and dietary patterns were verified using logistic regression analysis. Odds ratios (ORs) represented the probability of the adherence to tertiles of each dietary pattern. The reference groups (OR = 1.00) were those who declared that they did not follow the restrictions. Wald's test was used to assess the significance of ORs. Tests of linear trend across increasing tertiles of dietary pattern adherence (for ORs) were calculated for each type of eating restriction. P-value < 0.05 was considered as significant for all tests. All analyses were carried out applying sample weights to adjust for non-response and missing data. All analyses were performed using SAS 9.4. software (SAS Institute, Cary, NC, USA).

3. Results

3.1. Sample Characteristics

The sample consisted of 1007 participants (529 women and 478 men) aged 21 to 65 years. Among respondents, 35.7% were overweight and 12.7% were obese, that is their BMI calculated on the basis of declared height and weight was 25 and above. Table 1 displays characteristics of the study sample.

Table 1. Sample characteristics.

Variables		N = 1007	%
Gender	Female	529	52.5
	Male	478	47.5
Age	21–34 years	370	36.7
	35–44 years	235	23.3
	45–54 years	132	13.1
	55–65 years	270	26.8
Residence	City	539	53.5
	Town	199	19.8
	Country side	269	26.7
Education	Secondary and lower than secondary	403	40.1
	Higher	604	59.9
Body mass index (BMI) category	Underweight (BMI ≤ 18.5 kg/m^2)	35	3.5
	Normal weight (18.5 kg/m^2 < BMI ≤ 25 kg/m^2)	484	48.1
	Overweight (25 kg/m^2 < BMI ≤ 30 kg/m^2)	360	35.7
	Obesity (BMI > 30 kg/m^2)	128	12.7

N—number of participants

3.2. Dietary Patterns

The characteristics of the identified dietary patterns, i.e., 'Fruit and vegetables', 'Wholemeal food', 'Fast foods and sweets', 'Fruit and vegetable juices' and 'Meat and meat products', are summarized in Table 2 [28,29].

Table 2. Factor-loading matrix for the dietary patterns identified by principal component analysis (PCA).

Variables	Factor 1 Fast Foods and Sweets	Factor 2 Meat and Meat Products	Factor 3 Fruit and Vegetable	Factor 4 Whole Meal Food	Factor 5 Fruit and Vegetable Juices
Crisps and other salty snacks	0.824	.	.	.	.
Meals or snacks such as burgers, pizza, chicken, fries	0.756	.	.	.	.
Sweets and cakes	0.702	.	.	.	.
Fizzy drinks	0.633	.	.	.	.
Red meat (pork, beef, venison)	.	0.783	.	.	.
White meat (poultry, turkey)	.	0.748	.	.	.
Cured meats and sausages	.	0.696	.	.	.
Fried foods	.	0.551	.	.	.
Fruits	.	.	0.825	.	.
Vegetables	.	.	0.764	.	.
Cheeses (including melted cheese, blue cheese)	.	.	.	.	.
Whole meal pasta, groats	.	.	.	0.839	.
Whole meal bread	.	.	.	0.763	.
Fermented milk drinks	.	.	.	.	.
Vegetable juice	.	.	.	.	0.830
Fruit juice	.	.	.	.	0.799
Variance Explained (%)	24.9	16.0	9.5	7.4	6.4
Total Variance Explained (%)	64.2				
Kaiser's Measure of Sampling Adequacy:			0.781		

Factor loadings of ≤|0.50| are not shown in the table for simplicity.

3.3. Eating Restrictions

Nearly two-third (66.4%) of the study population declared following some restrictions in food consumption, of this 11.7% declared continuous use of the restrictions, and 54.7% occasional use.

The types of eating restrictions are described in Figure 1. Above two-fifths of the sample (42.4%) declared following restrictions regarding the quantity of consumed foods. In the total sample, the most common restrictions regarded consumption of sugar and/or sweets (47.6%), fats (24.9%), and high-fat foods (21.4%).

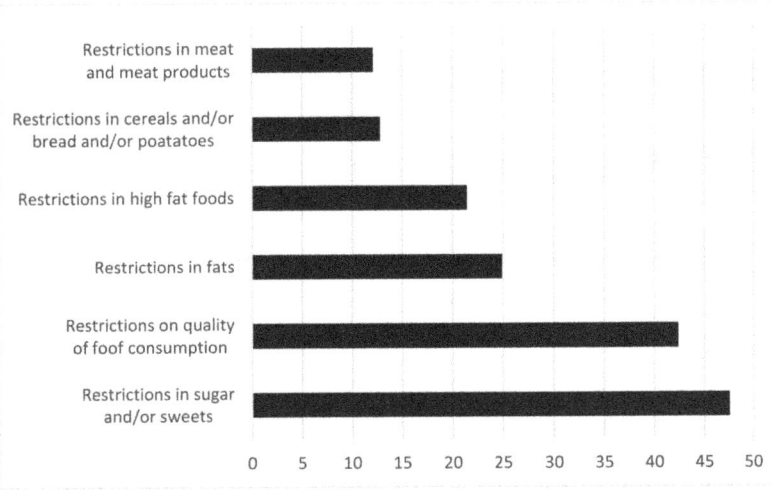

Figure 1. Eating restrictions in the sample (%).

3.4. Food Involvement

The mean value of the food involvement was 40.29, standard deviation—7.64 and median—40. The items included in the FIS are described in Table 3.

Table 3. Food Involvement Scale (FIS) characteristics.

Food Involvement Scale (FIS)	Mean	SD	Median
I think a lot about food each day.	3.01	1.02	3
Cooking or barbequing is a lot of fun.	3.55	1.01	4
Talking about what I ate or am going to eat is something I like to do.	3.27	1.03	3
Compared with other daily decisions, my food choices are very important.	2.67	1.04	3
When I travel, one of the things I anticipate most is eating the food there.	3.45	0.99	4
I do most or all of the clean up after eating.	3.66	0.93	4
I enjoy cooking for others and myself.	3.53	1.07	4
When I eat out, I think or talk a lot about how the food tastes.	3.27	0.98	3
I do like to mix or chop food.	3.28	1.07	3
I do most or all of my own food shopping.	3.44	1.16	4
I wash dishes or clean the table.	3.39	1.15	4
I care whether or not the table is nicely set.	7.74	0.90	4

SD—standard deviation.

3.5. Associations between Eating Restrictions, Food Involvement, and Dietary Patterns

The associations between variables are described in Tables 4 and 5. People in the upper tertile of 'Fruit and vegetables' compared to those in the bottom tertile of this DP were more likely to follow restrictions regarding quantity of consumed food (OR: 2.30, 95% confidence interval (CI) 1.66–3.19) and restrictions in consumption of sugar and/or sweets (OR: 1.89, 95% CI 1.36–2.61), fats (OR: 1.93, 95% CI 1.34–2.77), and high-fat foods (OR: 1.90, 95% CI 1.29–2.80). People in the upper tertile of 'Wholemeal food' compared to those in the bottom tertile of this DP were more likely to follow all included restrictions, i.e., restrictions regarding quantity of consumed food (OR: 1.76, 95% CI 1.27–2.45), restrictions in consumption of sugar and/or sweets (OR: 3.14, 95% CI 2.25–4.39), meat (OR: 3.13, 95% CI 1.83–5.35), fats (OR: 2.05, 95% CI 1.40–2.99), high-fat foods (OR: 1.78, 95% CI 1.20–2.65), and cereals and/or bread and/or potatoes (OR: 1.91, 95% CI 1.20–3.04).

People in the upper tertile of 'Meat and meat products' compared to those in the bottom tertile of this DP were less likely to follow restrictions in consumption of sugar and/or sweets (OR: 0.64, 95% CI 0.49–0.88), fats (OR: 0.68, 95% CI 0.47–0.98), high-fat foods (OR: 0.58, 95% CI 0.39–0.88) and meat (OR: 0.29, 95% CI 0.17–0.48). Whereas people in the upper tertile of 'Fast food and sweets' compared to those in the bottom tertile of this DP were less likely to follow all restrictions with exception of restriction in consumption of meat. Participants in the upper tertile of 'Fruit and vegetables juices' compared to those in the bottom tertile of this DP were less likely to follow restrictions regarding quantity of consumed food (OR: 0.61, 95% CI 0.44–0.85).

People in the upper tertiles of all DPs, with exception of 'Fast food and sweets', were more likely to be highly food involved compared to those in the bottom tertiles of these DPs. In the upper tertile of 'Wholemeal food' were more than threefold more likely to be highly food involved compared to the bottom tertile of this DP (more than 40 points in FIS) (Table 3).

Respondents who were highly food involved (FIS > 40 points) were more likely to declare restrictions in consumption of fats (OR: 1.35, 95% CI 1.01–1.80) and high-fat foods (OR: 1.64, 95% CI 1.21–2.23) (Table 4).

Table 4. Odds ratio (OR (95% confidence interval (CI)) of dietary patterns by eating restrictions in the sample.

Variable	Fast Foods and Sweets			Meat and Meat Products			Fruit and Vegetables			Whole Meal Food			Fruit and Vegetables Juices		
	T1	T3	p^a	T1	T3	p	T1	T3	p	T1	T3	p	T1	T3	p
Restriction on quantity of food consumption (ref.: without restrictions):															
OR crude (95%CI)	1	0.41 (0.30; 0.56)	****	1	0.94 (0.68; 1.30)	ns	1	2.30 (1.66; 3.19)	****	1	1.76 (1.27; 2.45)	***	1	0.61 (0.44; 0.85)	**
Restrictions in consumption of sugar and/or sweets (ref.: without restrictions):															
OR (95%CI)	1	0.35 (0.25; 0.48)	****	1	0.64 (0.49; 0.88)	***	1	1.89 (1.36; 2.61)	****	1	3.14 (2.25; 4.39)	****	1	0.88 (0.63; 1.22)	ns
Restrictions in consumption of fats (ref.: without restrictions):															
OR (95%CI)	1	0.42 (0.29; 0.61)	****	1	0.68 (0.47; 0.98)	*	1	1.93 (1.34; 2.77)	***	1	2.05 (1.40; 2.99)	***	1	0.89 (0.61; 1.28)	ns
Restrictions in consumption of high-fat foods (ref.: without restrictions):															
OR (95%CI)	1	0.23 (0.15; 0.36)	****	1	0.58 (0.39; 0.88)	***	1	1.90 (1.29; 2.80)	***	1	1.78 (1.20; 2.65)	**	1	1.13 (0.77; 1.67)	ns
Restrictions in consumption of cereals and/or bread and/or potatoes (ref.: without restrictions):															
OR (95%CI)	1	0.47 (0.30; 0.74)	****	1	1.16 (0.74; 1.83)	ns	1	0.80 (0.51; 1.27)	ns	1	1.91 (1.20; 3.04)	**	1	0.91 (0.57; 1.43)	ns
Restrictions in consumption of meat (ref.: without restrictions):															
OR (95%CI)	1	0.71 (0.44; 1.14)	ns	1	0.29 (0.17; 0.48)	****	1	1.32 (0.81; 2.15)	ns	1	3.13 (1.83; 5.35)	****	1	1.54 (0.94; 2.52)	ns
Food involvement (ref.: higher than 40 points)															
OR (95%CI)	1	1.30 (0.94; 1.79)	ns	1	1.80 (1.30; 2.49)	***	1	1.85 (1.34; 2.57)	***	1	3.46 (2.48; 4.82)	****	1	2.00 (1.44; 2.77)	****

^{a} statistically significant: * $p < 0.05$, ** $p < 0.01$, *** $p < 0.001$, **** $p < 0.0001$, ns—statistically insignificant (Wald's test); T1—the bottom tertile; T3—the upper tertile (T3—the most frequent consumption, while T1—the lowest consumption).

Table 5. Odds ratio (OR (95% CI) of food involvement by eating restrictions in Polish sample.

Eating Restrictions:	Food Involvement		
	FIS ≤ 40 Points	FIS > 40 Points	p^a
Restriction on quantity of food consumption (ref.: without restrictions):			
OR crude (95%CI)	1	1.06 (0.86; 1.42)	ns
Restrictions in consumption of sugar and/or sweets (ref.: without restrictions):			
OR (95%CI)	1	1.28 (0.96; 1.57)	ns
Restrictions in consumption of fats (ref.: without restrictions):			
OR (95%CI)	1	1.35 (1.01; 1.80)	*
Restrictions in consumption of high-fat foods (ref.: without restrictions):			
OR (95%CI)	1	1.64 (1.21; 2.23)	**
Restrictions in consumption of cereals and/or bread and/or potatoes (ref.: without restrictions):			
OR (95%CI)	1	1.32 (0.91; 1.92)	ns
Restrictions in consumption of meat (ref.: without restrictions):			
OR (95%CI)	1	1.27 (0.87; 1.86)	ns

[a] statistically significant: * $p < 0.05$, ** $p < 0.01$ ns—statistically insignificant (Wald's test); FIS—Food Involvement Scale score.

4. Discussion

The results of our study have shown that implementation of eating restrictions is a common practice, with over 60% of the participants reporting this behavior. Approximately 12% of respondents declared continuous use of restrictions in their diet. Thus, the results obtained in the group of Polish girls and young women [24] have been confirmed in the adults. It is a challenge for many individuals to practice dietary restriction, especially caloric restriction in an obesogenic environment so conducive to overeating [31]. A high percentage of people who declared restrictions points to the importance of this issue. Understanding the causes of these behaviors and their consequences for the diet should be deepened in further studies, especially since such practices are controversial. Eating restrictions may lead to unhealthy dietary habits and eating disorders [32]. On the other hand, moderate restraint in consumption of foods undesirable in a healthy diet and practising caloric restriction in the obesogenic environment could be considered as a beneficial and health promoting behavior [31].

Our findings have shown that restrictions in food quantity as well as those related to foods undesirable in a healthy diet (i.e., sugar, sweets, fats) were associated with healthy dietary patterns, mainly 'Fruit and vegetables' and 'Wholemeal food' DP. Participants who have reported restricting the overall quantity of food as well as sugar and/or sweets, fat, and foods high in fat adhered to the upper tertile of these DPs. Avoidance of foods high in fat and sugar by consumers who declared high intakes of fruit and vegetables has been previously reported [24,33]. Thus, this may be considered as evidence confirming the positive effects of food restrictions. Participants who restricted sugar and/or sweets and meat were more likely (approximately three times) to adhere to 'Wholemeal foods' DP, than those who restricted quantity of food, fats, high-fat foods, and starchy foods such as cereals, bread and potatoes. Because the awareness of the importance of a healthy lifestyle is increasing, breads containing whole grain, multi-grain, or functional components, such as fiber, attract attention of some consumers [34,35]. The higher health awareness of these people can explain their practices related to limiting sugar and/or sweets [36] and meat [37]. Restrictions regarding starchy foods in people from the upper tertile of 'Wholemeal foods' DP may result from using substitution of products originating from the refined flour (white bread, some cereals). Greater availability of wholemeal cereal products and the fact that these products meet more sensory expectations of consumers greatly facilitate such replacement [38].

Unhealthy dietary behaviors were found in participants from the upper tertile of 'Fast foods and sweets' DP, similarly to the research of Wadolowska et al. [39] carried out in young females. This may indicate the prevalence of this type of behavior in the Polish population, regardless of the age and gender. As expected, respondents with the highest adherence to this DP were less likely to restrict high-fat foods, sugar and sweets [24], but also fats and quantity of food. A lower tendency to limit consumption of such foods may indicate little or no interest in the quality of the diet and strong preferences for highly palatable foods. Similar results were obtained by French et al. [40] who found that higher frequency of fast foods consumption was more prevalent in women with low dietary restraint. Apart from low likelihood of restrictions in food quantity and foods rich in sugar and fat, in 'Fast foods and sweets' pattern we also observed a lower likelihood to restrict starchy foods such as cereals, bread and potatoes. In that context, absence of restrictions in unhealthy foods should be considered as a potential reason for excessive energy intake, especially because of the amount of energy, fat and sugar supplied with the diet. Many studies have linked low restraint with overweight and obesity [41,42].

Participants from the upper tertile of 'Meat and meat product' DP were less likely to restrict the consumption of majority of food products, mainly meat (by 71%), as well as fat (by 32%) and high-fat foods (by 42%). This finding confirms the similarity of food restrictions found for the "traditional Polish" pattern in the study of Galinski et al. [24]. Meat and meat dishes have always been and still are an important component of the traditional diet of Poles.

Dietary restrictions did not differentiate the probability of adherence to the upper tertile of the 'Fruit and vegetable juices' DP with one exception. Only in the case of restriction in food quantity, the adherence to the upper tertile of this DP was significantly lower compared to those from the bottom tertile (by 39%). Lack of restrictions may indicate a lack of behavioral control in a group of people who often drink juices. It may cause health risk because fruit juice is a source of sugar and low in fiber, which predisposes to weight gain and obesity [43], moreover drinking juice may replace eating fresh vegetables and fruits.

Frequent consumption of food characteristic for all DPs was more likely in people who were more food involved with one exception, the 'Fast food and sweets' DP. A higher intake of fruit and vegetables among individuals with a higher FIS was also reported by Marshall and Bell [14]. Nevertheless, by contrast with our research, they have found that highly food involved individuals were less likely to consume snack products. In our study people with higher food involvement were beyond threefold more likely to often consume wholemeal food compared to those in the bottom tertile of this DP which strongly confirms the relationship between food involvement and healthy diet. Nevertheless, our results only partially confirm that higher food involvement promotes more healthy diet [14] due to frequent consumption of meat and its products. This is also confirmed by the lack of a negative association with the consumption of fast food. Our results are, therefore, more consistent with those from the studies by Sarmugan and Worsley [16] who pointed out that consumers with higher levels of food involvement may be characterized by both healthier and less healthy dietary practices.

Nonetheless, participants who were more food involved (FIS > 40 points) were more likely to apply restrictions in fats and high-fat foods, which may be conducive to reducing energy intake. It is also confirmed by Marshall and Bell [14] who indicated that military personnel with higher FIS exhibited lower caloric intake, of which a lower proportion was derived from fat.

Most previous studies suggested that higher levels of food involvement appear to be associated with healthier dietary behavior [15,44] and we confirmed it partially. But it is also known that lower food involvement is associated with higher convenience orientation [45]. Because both the results of previous studies and of our research indicate some inconsistencies in relationship between food involvement and healthy food choices further research should be encouraged. Future studies should include also other factors conditioning food choice and eating behaviors, for example convenience which was not taken into account in our research.

The limitations of our study relate to the potential biases that may occur when self-reported data is analyzed. The most common biases in self-reported data are related to selective memory, telescoping, attribution, and exaggeration [46]. However, the main strength is a relatively large representative sample of the Polish population. The use of the questionnaire is also limited due to overestimation of some foods' consumption when Food Frequency Questionnaires (FFQ) is used. We have chosen FFQ because we aimed to see predominantly 'healthy' and 'unhealthy' dietary patterns, rather than exact amount of foods. Although our findings should not be generalized to the population with different cultural background, the study provides an interesting insight into dietary restrictions and their association with dietary patterns. The results can be used in the preparation of interventions targeted at health-related changes in existing dietary patterns.

5. Conclusions

Eating restrictions are a common practice among Poles, as they were used by over two thirds of the study sample. Declared restrictions in the consumption of foods high in sugar, fat and high-fat foods were observed in a group of people who often ate fruit, vegetable and wholemeal products. In addition, people who often consumed whole grains applied restrictions regarding eating meat and high-starch products. Such restrictions can be considered beneficial for health and interpreted as avoidance of foods that are not desirable in a healthy diet, especially when consumed in excess. There were no such restrictions in unhealthy dietary patterns, i.e., 'Fast foods and sweets' and Meat and meat products'. It could mean that the self-regulating behaviors do not occur among these adults. Further research should be focused on seeking explanations on why people who often eat sweets, fast food and meat are less likely to restrict less healthy food in their diet. It can be stated that dietary restrictions of sugar, high-fat foods and fats can be considered as predictors of healthy dietary patterns in the population of Polish adults.

Food involvement can be considered a factor that positively correlates with the use of food restrictions. However, participants with higher food involvement were more likely to use restrictions only regarding fats and high-fat foods, which may be conducive to reducing energy intake. Thus, higher level of food involvement appears to be associated with healthier dietary behavior. However, less healthy dietary practices may also be observed among more food-involved people, i.e., frequent consumption of meat. Some existing inconsistencies in relationship between food involvement and healthy food choices raise new questions, therefore further research should be encouraged. Future studies should include also other factors conditioning food choice and eating behaviors, for example convenience which was not taken into account in our research.

In conclusion, it should be stated that our assumption that individuals who are more food involved would be less able to use eating restrictions in comparison to less food-involved individuals was incorrect. Moreover, our results did not confirm that the dietary patterns of more food involved people are less healthy. We assumed that the intensity of the contact with food (high food involvement) encourages its consumption, and therefore makes it difficult to limit. The lack of confirmation of this assumption may suggest that food involvement associates rather with greater nutritional awareness, resulting in healthier dietary patterns in people who are more food involved. This may be relevant for creating public health policies: the combination of nutritional education with a greater personal commitment to learning about and experiencing food [47–49] could be more effective in inducing the change of diet to a healthier one.

Supplementary Materials: The following are available online at http://www.mdpi.com/2072-6643/12/4/1200/s1, Figure S1: Flow-chart of participants.

Author Contributions: All authors made substantial contributions to the design of the study, M.J.-Z. were involved in the data acquisition and wrote the manuscript; M.J.-Z. and J.G. analyzed and contributed to the interpretation of the data. All authors have read and agreed to the published version of the manuscript.

Funding: The research was financed by Polish Ministry of Science and Higher Education within funds of Faculty of Human Nutrition and Consumer Sciences, Warsaw University of Life Sciences (WULS), for scientific research. The publication of the article was financed by the Polish National Agency for Academic Exchange as part of the Foreign Promotion Program.

Acknowledgments: We express our sincere gratitude to the participants for contributions to the study.

Conflicts of Interest: The authors declare no conflict of interest.

References

1. Mond, J.; Van den Berg, P.; Boutelle, K.; Hannan, P.; Neumark-Sztainer, D. Obesity, body dissatisfaction, and emotional well-being in early and late adolescence: Findings from the project EAT study. *J. Adolesc. Heal.* **2011**, *48*, 373–378. [CrossRef]
2. Wardle, J.; Haase, A.M.; Steptoe, A.; Nillapun, M.; Jonwutiwes, K.; Bellisie, F. Gender differences in food choice: The contribution of health beliefs and dieting. *Ann. Behav. Med.* **2004**, *27*, 107–116. [CrossRef] [PubMed]
3. Fayet, F.; Petocz, P.; Samman, S. Prevalence and correlates of dieting in college women: A cross sectional study. *Int. J. Womens Health* **2012**, *4*, 405. [PubMed]
4. Iorga, M.; Manole, I.; Pop, L.; Muraru, I.-D.; Petrariu, F.-D. Eating disorders in relationship with dietary habits among pharmacy students in Romania. *Pharmacy* **2018**, *6*, 97. [CrossRef]
5. Kesse-Guyot, E.; Bertrais, S.; Peneau, S.; Estaquio, C.; Dauchet, L.; Vergnaud, A.C.; Czernichow, S.; Galan, P.; Hercberg, S.; Bellisle, F. Dietary patterns and their sociodemographic and behavioural correlates in French middle-aged adults from the SU. VI. MAX cohort. *Eur. J. Clin. Nutr.* **2009**, *63*, 521–528. [CrossRef] [PubMed]
6. Togo, P.; Osler, M.; Sørensen, T.I.A.; Heitmann, B.L. Food intake patterns and body mass index in observational studies. *Int. J. Obes.* **2001**, *25*, 1741–1751. [CrossRef]
7. Muñoz-Pareja, M.; Guallar-Castillón, P.; Mesas, A.E.; López-García, E.; Rodríguez-Artalejo, F. Obesity-related eating behaviors are associated with higher food energy density and higher consumption of sugary and alcoholic beverages: A cross-sectional study. *PLoS One* **2013**, *8*. [CrossRef]
8. *Diet, Nutrition, and the Prevention of Chronic Diseases: Report of a Joint WHO/FAO Expert Consultation*; WHO Technical Report Series 916; World Health Organization: Geneva, Switzerland, 2003; Volume 916.
9. Messier, S.P.; Mihalko, S.L.; Legault, C.; Miller, G.D.; Nicklas, B.J.; DeVita, P.; Beavers, D.P.; Hunter, D.J.; Lyles, M.F.; Eckstein, F. Effects of intensive diet and exercise on knee joint loads, inflammation, and clinical outcomes among overweight and obese adults with knee osteoarthritis: The IDEA randomized clinical trial. *Jama* **2013**, *310*, 1263–1273. [CrossRef]
10. Napoli, N.; Shah, K.; Waters, D.L.; Sinacore, D.R.; Qualls, C.; Villareal, D.T. Effect of weight loss, exercise, or both on cognition and quality of life in obese older adults. *Am. J. Clin. Nutr.* **2014**, *100*, 189–198. [CrossRef]
11. Bell, R.; Marshall, D.W. The construct of food involvement in behavioral research: Scale development and validation☆. *Appetite* **2003**, *40*, 235–244. [CrossRef]
12. Oliveros, E.; Somers, V.K.; Sochor, O.; Goel, K.; Lopez-Jimenez, F. The concept of normal weight obesity. *Prog. Cardiovasc. Dis.* **2014**, *56*, 426–433. [CrossRef] [PubMed]
13. Pliner, P.; Hobden, K. Development of a scale to measure the trait of food neophobia in humans. *Appetite* **1992**, *19*, 105–120. [CrossRef]
14. Marshall, D.; Bell, R. Relating the food involvement scale to demographic variables, food choice and other constructs. *Food Qual. Prefer.* **2004**, *15*, 871–879. [CrossRef]
15. Jarman, M.; Lawrence, W.; Ntani, G.; Tinati, T.; Pease, A.; Black, C.; Baird, J.; Barker, M.; Group, S.I.H.S. Low levels of food involvement and negative affect reduce the quality of diet in women of lower educational attainment. *J. Hum. Nutr. Diet.* **2012**, *25*, 444–452. [CrossRef] [PubMed]
16. Sarmugam, R.; Worsley, A. Dietary behaviours, impulsivity and food involvement: Identification of three consumer segments. *Nutrients* **2015**, *7*, 8036–8057. [CrossRef]
17. Olsen, S.O. Consumer involvement in seafood as family meals in Norway: An application of the expectancy-value approach. *Appetite* **2001**, *36*, 173–186. [CrossRef]
18. Juhl, H.J.; Poulsen, C.S. Antecedents and effects of consumer involvement in fish as a product group. *Appetite* **2000**, *34*, 261–267. [CrossRef]
19. Smith, A.D.A.C.; Emmett, P.M.; Newby, P.K.; Northstone, K. A comparison of dietary patterns derived by cluster and principal components analysis in a UK cohort of children. *Eur. J. Clin. Nutr.* **2011**, *65*, 1102. [CrossRef]
20. Ruano, C.; Henriquez, P.; Martínez-González, M.Á.; Bes-Rastrollo, M.; Ruiz-Canela, M.; Sanchez-Villegas, A. Empirically derived dietary patterns and health-related quality of life in the SUN project. *PLoS One* **2013**, *8*, e61490. [CrossRef]

21. Thorpe, M.G.; Milte, C.M.; Crawford, D.; McNaughton, S.A. A comparison of the dietary patterns derived by principal component analysis and cluster analysis in older Australians. *Int. J. Behav. Nutr. Phys. Act.* **2016**, *13*, 30. [CrossRef]
22. Esmaillzadeh, A.; Entezari, M.; Paknahad, Z.; Safavi, M.; Jalali, M.; Ghiasvand, R.; Bahreini, N.; Nourian, M.; Azadbakht, L. Identification of diet-disease relations through dietary pattern approach: A review. *J. Res. Med. Sci.* **2008**, *13*, 337–348.
23. Newby, P.K.; Tucker, K.L. Empirically derived eating patterns using factor or cluster analysis: A review. *Nutr. Rev.* **2004**, *62*, 177–203. [CrossRef] [PubMed]
24. Galinski, G.; Lonnie, M.; Kowalkowska, J.; Wadolowska, L.; Czarnocinska, J.; Jezewska-Zychowicz, M.; Babicz-Zielinska, E. Self-Reported Dietary Restrictions and Dietary Patterns in Polish Girls: A Short Research Report (GEBaHealth Study). *Nutrients* **2016**, *8*, 796. [CrossRef] [PubMed]
25. *Beliefs and Eating Habits Questionnaire. Behavioral Conditions of Nutrition Team, Committee of Human Nutrition Science*; Polish Academy of Science: Warsaw, Poland, 2014; Available online: http://www.knozc.pan.pl/ (accessed on 20 September 2017).
26. Kowalkowska, J.; Wadolowska, L.; Czarnocinska, J.; Czlapka-Matyasik, M.; Galinski, G.; Jezewska-Zychowicz, M.; Bronkowska, M.; Dlugosz, A.; Loboda, D.; Wyka, J. Reproducibility of a questionnaire for dietary habits, lifestyle and nutrition knowledge assessment (KomPAN) in Polish adolescents and adults. *Nutrients* **2018**, *10*, 1845. [CrossRef] [PubMed]
27. Field, A. *Discovering Statistics using IBM SPSS Statistics: North American Edition*; Sage: Thousand Oaks, CA, USA, 2017.
28. Jezewska-Zychowicz, M.; Gębski, J.; Guzek, D.; Świątkowska, M.; Stangierska, D.; Plichta, M.; Wasilewska, M. The Associations between Dietary Patterns and Sedentary Behaviors in Polish Adults (LifeStyle Study). *Nutrients* **2018**, *10*, 1004. [CrossRef] [PubMed]
29. Gębski, J.; Jezewska-Zychowicz, M.; Guzek, D.; Świątkowska, M.; Stangierska, D.; Plichta, M. The Associations between Dietary Patterns and Short Sleep Duration in Polish Adults (LifeStyle Study). *Int. J. Environ. Res. Public Health* **2018**, *15*, 2497. [CrossRef] [PubMed]
30. Cole, T.J.; Lobstein, T. Extended international (IOTF) body mass index cut-offs for thinness, overweight and obesity. *Pediatr. Obes.* **2012**, *7*, 284–294. [CrossRef]
31. Redman, L.M.; Ravussin, E. Caloric restriction in humans: Impact on physiological, psychological, and behavioral outcomes. *Antioxid. Redox Signal.* **2011**, *14*, 275–287. [CrossRef]
32. Nakai, Y.; Noma, S.; Nin, K.; Teramukai, S.; Wonderlich, S.A. Eating disorder behaviors and attitudes in Japanese adolescent girls and boys in high schools. *Psychiatry Res.* **2015**, *230*, 722–724. [CrossRef]
33. Ritchie, L.D.; Spector, P.; Stevens, M.J.; Schmidt, M.M.; Schreiber, G.B.; Striegel-Moore, R.H.; Wang, M.-C.; Crawford, P.B. Dietary patterns in adolescence are related to adiposity in young adulthood in black and white females. *J. Nutr.* **2007**, *137*, 399–406. [CrossRef]
34. Lyly, M.; Soini, E.; Rauramo, U.; Lähteenmäki, L. Perceived role of fibre in a healthy diet among Finnish consumers. *J. Hum. Nutr. Diet.* **2004**, *17*, 231–239. [CrossRef] [PubMed]
35. Mialon, V.S.; Clark, M.R.; Leppard, P.I.; Cox, D.N. The effect of dietary fibre information on consumer responses to breads and "English" muffins: A cross-cultural study. *Food Qual. Prefer.* **2002**, *13*, 1–12. [CrossRef]
36. Lee, Y.; Joo, N. The awareness level and needs for education on reducing sugar consumption among mothers with preschool children. *Nutr. Res. Pract.* **2016**, *10*, 229–236. [CrossRef] [PubMed]
37. Kayser, M.; Nitzko, S.; Spiller, A. Analysis of differences in meat consumption patterns. *Int. Food Agribus. Manag. Rev.* **2013**, *16*, 43–56.
38. Adams, J.F.; Engstrom, A. Dietary intake of whole grain vs. recommendations. *Cereal Foods World* **2000**, *45*, 75–78.
39. Wadolowska, L.; Kowalkowska, J.; Lonnie, M.; Czarnocinska, J.; Jezewska-Zychowicz, M.; Babicz-Zielinska, E. Associations between physical activity patterns and dietary patterns in a representative sample of Polish girls aged 13-21 years: A cross-sectional study (GEBaHealth Project). *BMC Public Health* **2016**, *16*, 1–14. [CrossRef]
40. French, S.A.; Harnack, L.; Jeffery, R.W. Fast food restaurant use among women in the Pound of Prevention study: Dietary, behavioral and demographic correlates. *Int. J. Obes.* **2000**, *24*, 1353–1359. [CrossRef]
41. Burton, P.; Smit, H.J.; Lightowler, H.J. The influence of restrained and external eating patterns on overeating. *Appetite* **2007**, *49*, 191–197. [CrossRef]

42. Ernst, B.; Wilms, B.; Thurnheer, M.; Schultes, B. Eating behaviour in treatment-seeking obese subjects–Influence of sex and BMI classes. *Appetite* **2015**, *95*, 96–100. [CrossRef]
43. Hebden, L.; O'Leary, F.; Rangan, A.; Singgih Lie, E.; Hirani, V.; Allman-Farinelli, M. Fruit consumption and adiposity status in adults: A systematic review of current evidence. *Crit. Rev. Food Sci. Nutr.* **2017**, *57*, 2526–2540. [CrossRef]
44. Barker, M.; Lawrence, W.; Woadden, J.; Crozier, S.R.; Skinner, T.C. Women of lower educational attainment have lower food involvement and eat less fruit and vegetables. *Appetite* **2008**, *50*, 464–468. [CrossRef] [PubMed]
45. Candel, M.J.J.M. Consumers' convenience orientation towards meal preparation: Conceptualization and measurement. *Appetite* **2001**, *36*, 15–28. [CrossRef] [PubMed]
46. Brutus, S.; Aguinis, H.; Wassmer, U. Self-reported limitations and future directions in scholarly reports: Analysis and recommendations. *J. Manage.* **2013**, *39*, 48–75. [CrossRef]
47. Burton, M.; Reid, M.; Worsley, A.; Mavondo, F. Food skills confidence and household gatekeepers' dietary practices. *Appetite* **2017**, *108*, 183–190. [CrossRef] [PubMed]
48. Begley, A.; Paynter, E.; Butcher, L.M.; Dhaliwal, S.S. Effectiveness of an Adult Food Literacy Program. *Nutrients* **2019**, *11*, 797. [CrossRef] [PubMed]
49. Rathi, N.; Riddell, L.; Worsley, A. Secondary school students' views of food and nutrition education in Kolkata, India. *Health Educ.* **2017**, *117*, 310–322. [CrossRef]

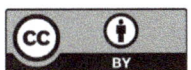

© 2020 by the authors. Licensee MDPI, Basel, Switzerland. This article is an open access article distributed under the terms and conditions of the Creative Commons Attribution (CC BY) license (http://creativecommons.org/licenses/by/4.0/).

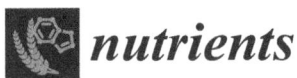

Article

Traditional Dietary Patterns and Risk of Mortality in a Longitudinal Cohort of the Salus in Apulia Study

Roberta Zupo [1], Rodolfo Sardone [1,*], Rossella Donghia [2], Fabio Castellana [1], Luisa Lampignano [1], Ilaria Bortone [1], Giovanni Misciagna [1], Giovanni De Pergola [3], Francesco Panza [1,4], Madia Lozupone [1,4], Andrea Passantino [5], Nicola Veronese [6], Vito Guerra [2], Heiner Boeing [2,7] and Gianluigi Giannelli [8]

1. Population Health Unit —"Salus in Apulia Study"—National Institute of Gastroenterology "Saverio de Bellis", Research Hospital, Castellana Grotte, 70013 Bari, Italy; zuporoberta@gmail.com (R.Z.); castellanafabio@hotmail.it (F.C.); luisalampignano@gmail.com (L.L.); ilariabortone@gmail.com (I.B.); gmisciagn@libero.it (G.M.); f_panza@hotmail.com (F.P.); madia.lozupone@gmail.com (M.L.)
2. Data Analysis Unit, National Institute of Gastroenterology "Saverio de Bellis", Research Hospital, Castellana Grotte, 70013 Bari, Italy; rossydonghia@gmail.com (R.D.); vito.guerra@irccsdebellis.it (V.G.); boeing@dife.de (H.B.)
3. Clinical Nutrition Unit, Medical Oncology, Department of Biomedical Science and Human Oncology, University of Bari, School of Medicine, Policlinico, Piazza Giulio Cesare 11, 70124 Bari, Italy; gdepergola@libero.it
4. Neurodegenerative Disease Unit, Department of Basic Medicine, Neuroscience, and Sense Organs, University of Bari Aldo Moro, 70121 Bari, Italy
5. Department of Cardiology and Cardiac Rehabilitation, Scientific Clinical Institutes Maugeri, IRCCS Institute of Cassano Murge, 70020 Bari, Italy; andrea.passantino@icsmaugeri.it
6. Azienda ULSS 3 Serenissima, Primary Care Department, District 3, 30174 Venice, Italy; ilmannato@gmail.com
7. German Institute of Human Nutrition Potsdam-Rehbrücke, 14558 Nuthetal, Germany
8. Scientific direction, National Institute of Gastroenterology "Saverio de Bellis", Research Hospital, Castellana Grotte, 70013 Bari, Italy; gianluigi.giannelli@irccsdebellis.it
* Correspondence: rodolfo.sardone@irccsdebellis.it; Tel.: +39-080-4994662

Received: 10 March 2020; Accepted: 10 April 2020; Published: 12 April 2020

Abstract: There is still room for further studies analyzing the long-term health impact of specific dietary patterns observable in regions belonging to the Mediterranean area. The aim of the study is to evaluate how much a diet practiced in southern Italy is associated to a risk of mortality. The study population included 2472 participants first investigated in 1985, inquiring about their frequencies of intake of 29 foods using a self-administered questionnaire covering the previous year. The population was followed up for mortality until 31 December 2017. Cox-based risk modeling referred to single foods, food groups, the results of principal component analysis (PCA), and a priori indexes. Single food analysis revealed eggs, fatty meat, and fatty/baked ham to be inversely associated with mortality. Furthermore, one of the 5 PCA derived dietary patterns, the "Farmhouse" pattern, showed a higher hazard ratio (HR), mostly driven by dairy products. In subsequent analyses, the increased risk of mortality for fresh cheese and decreased risk for fatty ham and eggs were confirmed. The a priori diet indexes (Italian Meddiet, Meddietscore, Dietary Approaches to Stop Hypertension (DASH), and Mediterranean–DASH Intervention for Neurodegenerative Delay diet (MIND) indexes) showed borderline inverse relationships. In a Mediterranean population with an overall healthy diet, foods such as eggs and fatty meat, reflecting dietary energy and wealth, played a role in prolonging the life of individuals. Our study confirms that some dairy products might have a detrimental role in mortality in the Mediterranean setting.

Keywords: healthy diet indexes; food intake; apulia; mind index; dash index; med-diet score

1. Introduction

In the last decades, life expectancy has increased in most parts of the world and population aging is now a global phenomenon, especially in developed countries. In Europe, the life expectancy of the Italian population is the second highest, being two years longer than the European average, based on a gain of 2.8 years in life expectancy between 2000 to 2015. However, this advantage of the Italian population in terms of life expectancy compared to their other European peers is not reflected in a similar gain in disability-free years, as reported by the Institute for Health Metrics and Evaluation (IHME).

This relatively privileged situation in terms of life expectancy in Italy might be related to the lifestyle, in particular, the diet consumed in this country. Meta-analyses with mortality as endpoint identified a number of food groups making up the Italian diet that are associated with a reduced risk of mortality, such as high intake of vegetables, fruits, fish, legumes, nuts, and whole grains, and a low intake of red and processed meat [1–4]. Accordingly, dietary indexes defined a priori, including those foods such as the Mediterranean-Diet score [5], the Healthy Eating index [6], the Alternate Healthy Eating index [7], or the Dietary Approaches to Stop Hypertension index (DASH) [8], were found to be associated with a reduced risk of all-cause mortality.

The dietary pattern in Italy is the heritage of millennia of exchanges of people, cultures, and foods among all countries around the Mediterranean basin, ever since the Greek and Roman expansions. This diet is rich in plant foods (cereals, fruit, vegetables, nuts, and legumes), with olive oil as the principal source of added fat, combined with a moderate intake of animal foods, including dairy products, and drinking wine especially during meals [9,10].

Fortunately, there are areas in Italy where the traditional Italian diet is still practiced by a large part of the population. Recently, we confirmed that the local population of Castellana Grotte, located in Apulia, has shown a very stable dietary behavior over the past years (Castellana et al. 2019), despite some changes in the last decades [11]. In this town and other parts of Italy, most of the foods are produced locally, such as fruits, vegetables, and legumes. In addition, the Apulian diet includes specific regional varieties such as orecchiette as the main pasta, and the bread is produced with semolina flour, an unrefined type of flour with a rich dietary fiber content (Castellana et al. 2019).

The long tradition of research into diet, launched by the National Institute of Gastroenterology "S. De Bellis" (IRCCS) with the establishment of a prospective cohort study in 1985, involving more than 2500 participants from Castellana Grotte, a small town south of Bari and the seat of the Institute, allowed investigation of the long-term role of food intake for risk of mortality to be investigated in a Mediterranean diet setting. The risk modeling included the investigation of single foods, food groups, the results of principal component analysis (PCA), and *a priori* healthy diet indexes.

2. Materials and Methods

2.1. Study Population:

In the beginning of the 1980s, the IRCCS De Bellis participated in the Multicenter Italian study on Cholelithiasis (MICOL) [12] with the aim of prospectively investigating the role of lifestyle and nutrition in gastrointestinal and other chronic diseases, including cholelithiasis [13,14]. In 1985, a random sample of 3500 subjects (2000 men and 1500 women) aged ≥30 years was drawn from the electoral roll of Castellana Grotte (17,334 residents at the 1981 census); 2472 (1429 men and 1043 women) agreed to participate (70.6% response rate). Thus, the study population could be considered as a representative sample of the population of Puglia of that time (1980s). The cohort was reexamined several times over the past three decades (Castellana et al. 2019). In the current investigation, we took into account only the first survey in 1985 (M1) with a follow-up on mortality until 31 December 2017. The mortality data were obtained from the Electronic Health Records of the Regione Puglia. All participants agreed to take part in the MICOL study, giving informed consent and allowing sharing of their medical data, including the death events and causes of death, with the study team. All study procedures were in accordance with the ethical standards of the institutional research committee and with the 1964 Helsinki declaration. Every single examination and informed consent form was approved by the Institutional Review Board of the National Institute of Gastroenterology and Research Hospital. All study information is stored in electronic databases that are protected according to Italian privacy laws.

2.2. Dietary and Lifestyle Variables

A self-administered ad hoc questionnaire was provided by the MICOL Group and assessed dietary habits of the previous year. In the questionnaire, the intakes of 29 foods were inquired about as frequencies per week in categories from 0 to 4 (0 = never, 1= rarely, 2 = occasionally, 3 = frequently, 4 = daily). Separately from foods, the use of olive oil was assessed in three categories (0 = never, 1 = occasionally, 2 = frequently) and the consumption of wine in six categories ranging from 0 consumption to more than 2 L a day. The self-administered questionnaire was checked for completeness by a physician during an interview at the study center. The interview was conducted by a medical doctor and included questions on lifestyle aspects such as educational level, physical activity, and smoking. Additionally, at the interview, anthropometric data were obtained, such as weight (kg) and height (cm), measured with SECA 700 and SECA 220 (Seca GmBH and Co., Hamburg, Germany), from which the body mass index (BMI) was derived, calculated as the ratio of weight (kg) to height squared (m^2). Multimorbidity status was defined as the co-presence of two or more chronic diseases measured by the presence of the following conditions: diabetes, hypertension, peptic ulcer, cholangiolithiasis, myocardial infarction, hepatic cirrhosis or other liver diseases, inflammatory bowel diseases, major infectious diseases, leukemia or other blood chronic diseases, viral hepatitis, AIDS [15]. All diseases were assessed using a general medical history questionnaire administered by an expert physician.

2.3. Food Group and Dietary Patterns

2.3.1. Food Groups

Food groups were formed by summarizing the frequencies of single foods such as legumes (peas, beans, lentils, fava beans, chickpeas), vegetables (raw and cooked vegetables), fresh cheese (sheep and cow ricotta, fiordilatte, mozzarella, smoked provola, and other cheese), red meat (low-fat meat and fatty meat), processed meat (cotechino, zampone, cured meat, sausages, lean ham, fatty ham), fish and seafood (e.g., mussels, tuna, oysters, salmon), and sweets (croissant, buns, and chocolate).

2.3.2. A Priori Dietary Pattern

Four healthy/preventive diet indexes were calculated according to published algorithms that were adapted to the available food information: Meddiet score [16], DASH-diet index [8], MIND-diet index [17], and Italian Meddiet index [18]. Each index was created by defining the dietary components that contributed to the index, adding the frequencies of the foods contributing to the components, and using the median value of the total sample as the cut-off, if not otherwise instructed.

2.3.3. A Posteriori Dietary Patterns

A robust algorithm of data reduction, the PCA [19], was applied to the 29 food frequencies to summarize new variables, such as principal components, that we defined as new dietary patterns. We selected the first five principal components according to the "percentage of variance" criterion; this means that the cumulative percentage (eigenvalue x 100) of variance explained from the components 1 to 5 covered 95% of the information. Subsequently, two trained nutritionists (L.L. and F.C.) interpreted the PCA components and agreed on a proper naming of the pattern. The naming was approved by a third senior nutritionist (R.Z.).

2.3.4. Predictive Variables for the Outcomes

In order to select the most predictive foods for mortality, we used a machine-learning algorithm, the random survival forest (RSF) [20]. This algorithm was able to select the best predictor in a set of 29 variables. The latter were filtered using variable importance criterion (VIMP): large importance values indicated variables with higher predictive power. Furthermore, to better improve the data output interpretation of RSF, we implemented an automated backward elimination procedure; this represents a corroborated method for highly correlated complex data, to avoid noise in data outputs [21].

2.3.5. Mortality Assessment

In order to explore the association of dietary patterns and foods on cause-specific mortality, we categorized findings on the basis of three different causes. Firstly, death for all-causes, secondly deaths subsequent to all types of cancers, finally, deaths due to cardiovascular and cerebrovascular diseases (mostly strokes and myocardial infarction). All causes were taken from the Apulia Region Public Health Records, assessed using International Classification of Diseases (ICD)-10 classification. We limited the investigation to the most common causes of death because they provide enough cases to run the Cox proportion models.

2.4. Statistical Analysis

Data are reported as means ± standard deviations (M ± SD) for continuous measures, and frequency and percentages (%) for all categorical variables. We used Cox modeling to explore the relationship between overall and specific-cause mortality and explanatory variables, estimating the hazard rate ratio (HR) and 95% confidence interval (95% CI). The HR was taken as an approximation of the relative risk (RR). Each subject was censored by the end of follow-up (31 December 2017), the date of death or the date of termination of study participation. For Cox modeling of the food variables, the following covariates as potential risk factors, were used: age (continuous variable), sex (dichotomous variable), BMI (continuous variable), educational level (categorized as no schooling, primary school, secondary school/university degree), smoking (categorized as never-smoker and former smoker/current smoker (≤20 cigarettes/d and >20 cigarettes/d), multimorbidity (two categories: >2 and <2 prevalent diseases), wine (categorized as non-consumer and consumer of less than 1 L and more than 1 L a day), and olive oil (categorized as frequent users and less frequent users).

Various statistical approaches were used to identify the food groups associated with mortality. Firstly, the 29 food groups were related to mortality, adjusted for covariates (see above). Significant results according to the 95% CI are highlighted in bold in the table. These food groups were further used in a multiple Cox regression model applying the backward stepwise method. Only variables that showed associations with $p < 0.10$ were left in the models. The foods selected in such a way were related to mortality, mutually adjusted, and the variables that showed associations with $p < 0.10$ were left in the models. In further approaches, it was investigated whether food groups related to a risk of mortality, in the initial analysis with covariates, still dominated the results regarding the outcome mortality. One approach was to form broader food groups and relate these groups to mortality. Other approaches were of a more exploratory nature. The a priori (Meddiet score, DASH, and MIND index) and a posteriori (PCA) food patterns were related to a risk of mortality. Furthermore, the foods most predictive of the RSF were also related to the outcome. Finally, we related the foods associated with mortality also to cause-specific mortality. All analyses were performed using StataCorp 2017 Stata (Release 15 statistical software, College Station, TX, StataCorp LLC).

3. Results

Baseline characteristics of the M1 cohort population are presented in Table 1. These variables were also selected as confounders for the risk modeling of the dietary variables and hence, also yielded the mutually adjusted hazard ratio (HR). The M1 population was nearly balanced regarding gender, with a slight dominance of men, was middle-aged, being about 50 years old on average, most had low education, featuring 5 years of schooling or less, and obese according to the traditional classification of BMI. Smoking was not widespread for the time period of the mid-1980s to 1990s, compared to other populations, and was more common among men (45.7% men and 12.8% women). Drinking more than one liter per day of wine showed a clear dominance among men compared to women (19.1% against 1.5%). Olive oil dominated as a fat source and one-third declared frequent use.

Table 1. Baseline characteristics of MICOL 1 subjects ($n = 2472$) and associated hazard ratios, adjusted for age and sex, and mutually adjusted.

Variables	Frequencies *	HR of Mortality Mutually Adjusted (95% CI)
Gender (Female) (%)	1043 (42.19)	0.65 (0.56 to 0.75)
Age (yrs) (M±SD)	48.00 ± 10.71	1.12 (1.11 to 1.13)
Education (%)		
Low (≤ 5years)	1657 (67.03)	1
Medium (8 years)	457 (18.49)	0.95 (0.79 to 1.16)
High (> 8years)	358 (14.48)	0.89 (0.70 to 1.13)
Smoking (%)	788 (31.88)	1.63 (1.40 to 1.89)
Body Mass Index (kg/m^2)	27.48±4.55	1.04 (1.02 to 1.05)
Wine (≥ 1 lt/day) (%)	289 (11.69)	0.96 (0.79 to 1.16)
Comorbidity (≥ 2) (%)	154 (6.23)	1.20 (0.97 to 1.49)
Frequent use of olive oil (%)	864 (34.95)	0.84 (0.73 to 0.96)

* Proportion for categorical and means and standard deviation for continuous variables.

Of the 2472 participants, 990 died. This equals 400 deaths per one million person years. Cox regression modeling revealed a reduced risk of mortality for females and for a frequent use of olive oil. Increased risks were found for age, smoking, and body mass index. All estimates were in line with current knowledge about lifestyle factors that influence the risk of mortality.

The frequency information covered 29 food items. The mean frequencies—expressed as consumption per day—are shown for the total group and for men and women (Table 2). The frequencies of semolina type bread and fruit stood out, showing a frequency of several times per day. Raw and cooked vegetables were eaten every second day, alternating with legumes. Consumption of milk and dairy products such as ricotta or mozzarella was widespread (Table 2). Intake of men and women did not differ in principle in terms of frequency, allowing a combined analysis across gender. The main difference between gender regarded semolina type bread eaten by men compared to women (+0.07 per day), followed by desserts (−0.04), fatty meat (+0.04), skimmed milk (−0.04), sheep ricotta (−0.04), cow ricotta (−0.04), and raw and cooked vegetables (−0.04).

According to the percentage of variance, we selected the first five components as food patterns consumed by the Castellana population. The 5 food patterns are shown in Figure 1 Figure 2 Figure 3 Figure 4 Figure 5. The first food pattern (Figure 1) reflected high frequencies, particularly of cured meat, sausages, lean ham, and bacon, followed by desserts, chocolate, and packaged/fried foods. It was named the "Energy-Rich Foods Pattern". The second food pattern (Figure 2) reflected a high-frequency intake of all dairy products, including fresh and other cheeses, integrated in a diet with a lot of vegetables, legumes, fruits, and semolina type bread. It was named the "Farmhouse Diet". The third food pattern (Figure 3) reflected a high frequency of intake of sweets such as desserts, chocolate, and package products. It was named the "Sweets Pattern". The fourth food pattern (Figure 4) reflected a high frequency of intake of whole grains, poultry, fish, seafood, and legumes. It was named the "Winter Pattern". The fifth food pattern (Figure 5) reflected a high consumption of whole milk, semolina type bread, legumes, and vegetables. It was named the "Elderly Pattern".

Table 2. Foods from the questionnaire, expressed as frequency per day.

Foods	Total Sample (M ± SD)	Men (M ± SD)	Women (M ± SD)
Whole grain bread (Pane integrale)	0.09 ± 0.34	0.08 ± 0.32	0.11 ± 0.37
Semolina type and other bread (Pane bianco)	1.28 ± 0.66	1.31 ± 0.65	1.24 ± 0.67
Pasta, rice, polenta (Pasta, riso, polenta)	0.52 ± 0.26	0.53 ± 0.26	0.50 ± 0.25
Desserts (Torte, crostate)	0.17 ± 0.17	0.16 ± 0.16	0.20 ± 0.18
Low-fat meat (Carne magra)	0.34 ± 0.11	0.35 ± 0.11	0.34 ± 0.11
Fatty meat (Carne di maiale)	0.12 ± 0.14	0.13 ± 0.14	0.09 ± 0.14
Poultry, rabbit (Pollame e coniglio)	0.25 ± 0.15	0.25 ± 0.15	0.25 ± 0.15
Cotechino, zampone (Cotechino, zampone)	0.005 ± 0.033	0.005 ± 0.03	0.006 ± 0.04
Cured meat, sausages (Salumi, salsiccia)	0.13 ± 0.15	0.14 ± 0.15	0.11 ± 0.15
Lean ham (Prosciutto magro)	0.13 ± 0.14	0.14 ± 0.15	0.12 ± 0.14
Fatty ham, ham (Prosciutto grasso o cotto)	0.13 ± 0.14	0.14 ± 0.14	0.13 ± 0.14
Bacon, cheek lard (Pancetta e guanciale)	0.04 ± 0.07	0.04 ± 0.08	0.03 ± 0.07
Meat sauce (Sughi di carne, ragù)	0.32 ± 0.12	0.33 ± 0.12	0.32 ± 0.11
Fish (Pesce)	0.23 ± 0.15	0.23 ± 0.15	0.23 ± 0.15
Seafoods (Frutti di mare)	0.07 ± 0.10	0.07 ± 0.12	0.06 ± 0.08
Whole milk (Latte intero)	0.25 ± 0.45	0.25 ± 0.45	0.26 ± 0.45
Skimmed milk, low fat milk (Latte scremato o parzialmente scremato)	0.26 ± 0.44	0.24 ± 0.43	0.28 ± 0.46
Sheep ricotta, fiordilatte, mozzarella, smoked provola (Ricotta di pecora, fiordilatte, mozzarella, provola affumicata)	0.29 ± 0.18	0.27 ± 0.19	0.31 ± 0.16
Cow ricotta (Ricotta di vacca)	0.15 ± 0.15	0.13 ± 0.14	0.17 ± 0.15
Other cheeses (Altri formaggi)	0.27 ± 0.18	0.27 ± 0.19	0.27 ± 0.18
Eggs (Uova)	0.20 ± 0.16	0.19 ± 0.16	0.20 ± 0.16
Fried foods (Alimenti fritti)	0.18 ± 0.15	0.19 ± 0.15	0.18 ± 0.15
Chocolate (Cioccolata)	0.07 ± 0.12	0.06 ± 0.13	0.07 ± 0.12
Croissant, buns, pizzas (cornetti, maritozzi, pizza)	0.04 ± 0.11	0.04 ± 0.13	0.03 ± 0.10
Typical local rotisserie (Supplì, calzone, arancini)	0.08 ± 0.09	0.08 ± 0.10	0.08 ± 0.09
Sandwiches (Tramezzini)	0.01 ± 0.06	0.02 ± 0.07	0.01 ± 0.04
Legumes: peas, beans, lentils, fava beans, chickpeas (Legumi: piselli, fagioli, lenticchie, fave, ceci)	0.32 ± 0.11	0.32 ± 0.11	0.31 ± 0.12
Raw vegetables, Cooked vegetables (Verdure crude e cotte)	0.41 ± 0.23	0.39 ± 0.23	0.43 ± 0.24
Fresh fruit (Frutta fresca)	1.81 ± 0.50	1.76 ± 0.55	1.88 ± 0.40

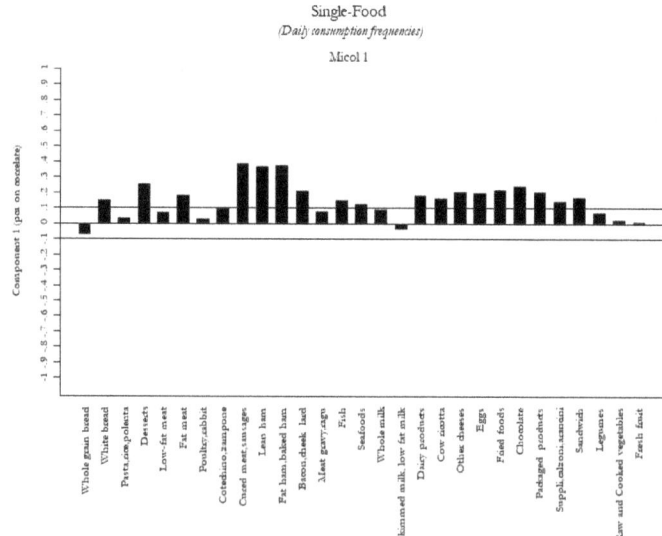

Figure 1. First dietary pattern, "Energy-Rich Foods Pattern", derived with principal component analysis.

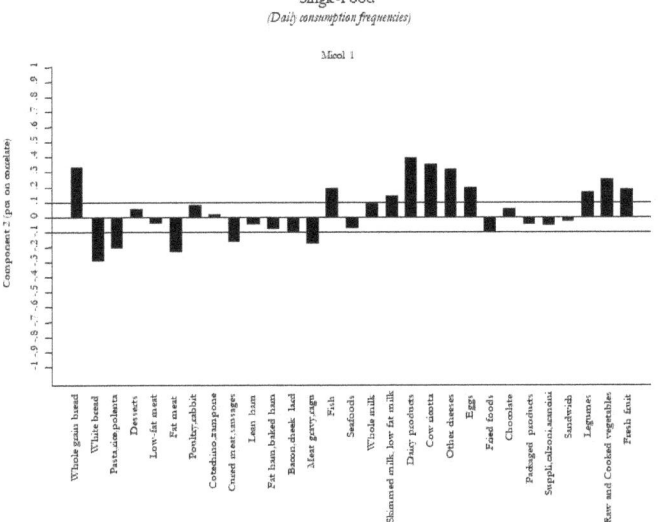

Figure 2. Second dietary pattern "Farmhouse Diet" derived with principal component analysis.

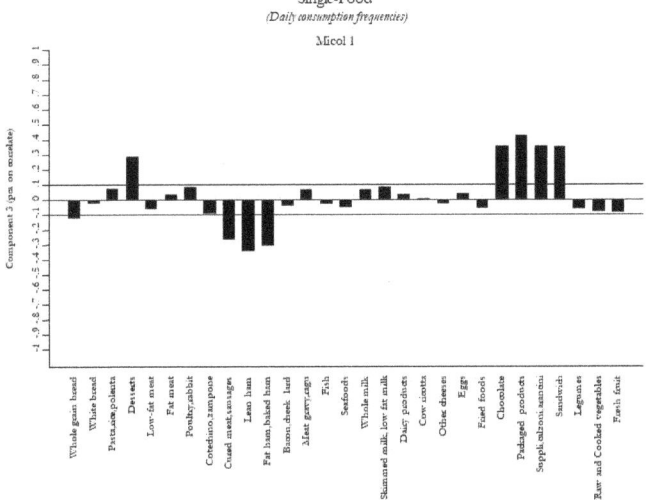

Figure 3. Third dietary pattern, "Sweets Pattern", derived with principal component analysis.

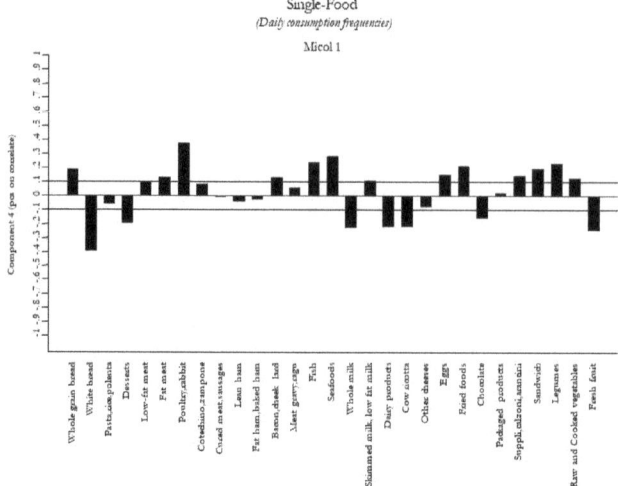

Figure 4. Fourth dietary pattern, "Winter Pattern", derived with principal component analysis.

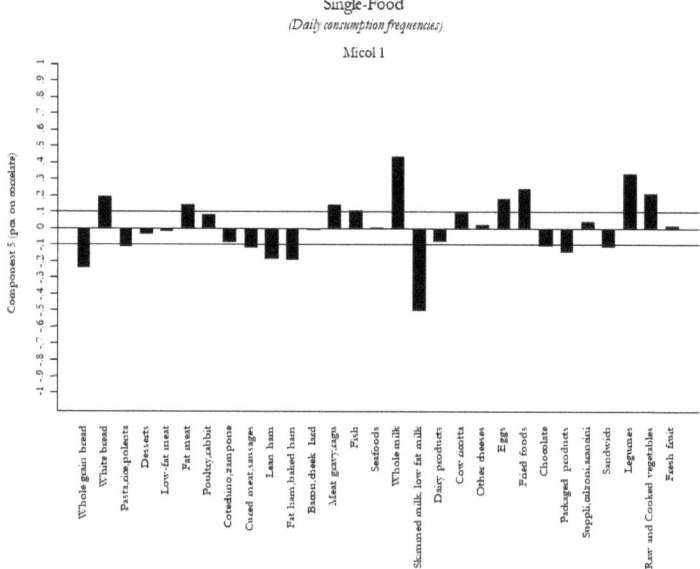

Figure 5. Fifth dietary pattern, "Elderly Pattern", derived with principal component analysis

In Table 3, the hazard ratios (HR) for mortality for intake of food per week are shown. Only a few food items were significantly related to risk; this did not include the obvious candidates such as fruit and vegetables. Instead, fatty meat, fatty/baked ham, and eggs showed an inverse relationship between frequency and risk of mortality. Further suggestive but non-significant relations were seen for semolina type bread (inverse), and sheep ricotta, mozzarella, smoked provola (positive).

Table 3. Cox regression model of mortality for foods (per one frequency per day) in the questionnaire, adjusted for covariates *.

Foods in Questionnaire	HR of Mortality for one Frequency Per Day, Adjusted for Covariates (95% CI)
Whole grain bread	1.10 (0.93 to 1.30)
Semolina type band other bread	0.92 (0.83 to 1.02)
Pasta, rice, polenta	0.92 (0.71 to 1.18)
Desserts	0.89 (0.58 to 1.37)
Low-fat meat	0.86 (0.48 to 1.53)
Fatty meat	**0.60 (0.37 to 0.99)**
Poultry, rabbit	1.02 (0.67 to 1.54)
Cotechino, zampone	0.16 (0.01 to 2.07)
Cured meat, sausages	0.78 (0.47 to 1.28)
Lean ham	0.82 (0.50 to 1.35)
Fatty ham, ham	**0.59 (0.35 to 0.99)**
Bacon, cheek lard	0.72 (0.25 to 2.09)
Meat sauce	1.55 (0.85 to 2.82)
Fish	0.80 (0.53 to 1.22)
Seafood	0.63 (0.33 to 1.22)
Whole milk	1.07 (0.93 to 1.23)
Skimmed milk, low-fat milk	1.00 (0.87 to 1.15)
Sheep ricotta, fiordilatte, mozzarella, smoked provola	**1.36 (0.99 to 1.86)**
Cow ricotta	1.45 (0.94 to 2.24)
Other cheeses	1.05 (0.73 to 1.52)
Eggs	**0.63 (0.42 to 0.95)**
Fried foods	1.11 (0.72 to 1.71)
Chocolate	1.05 (0.56 to 1.97)
Croissant, buns, pizzas	0.55 (0.24 to 1.27)
Typical local rotisserie	0.89 (0.42 to 1.87)
Sandwiches	0.79 (0.16 to 3.75)
Legumes: peas, beans, lentils, fava beans, chickpeas	1.17 (0.68 to 2.01)
Raw vegetables, cooked vegetables	1.06 (0.80 to 1.41)
Fresh fruit	1.00 (0.88 to 1.15)

Statistical significance is represented in bold. * Model corrected for sex (male, female), age (yrs), BMI (unit), education (low, medium, high), smoking (yes, no), comorbidity (≥2 vs. <2), wine (≥1 L/day vs. <1 L/day), olive oil, (extensive use vs. non-extensive use).

In the first lines of Table 4, the HRs for the combined frequencies reflecting food groups are shown. This analysis now showed a significantly increased risk with increased frequency of ricotta type cheese, and some but non-significant suggestions that processed meat in general was associated with a reduced risk. The previous risk analyses of foods did not include the adjustment for other foods, which is in line with the exploratory nature of the study. The role of such adjustments was investigated via backward selection, starting from a fully adjusted model. The result with the first five foods is shown in Table 4. It appeared that only two (fatty/baked ham, eggs) of the three in the unadjusted risk models for other foods identified foods (fat meat, fatty/baked ham, eggs) were still related to risk but sheep ricotta, previously suggestively related to risk, now reached significance. The fifth food analyzed with the backward approach did not reach significance at the 5% level.

The role of dietary variables was also investigated by random survival forest (RSF), a machine learning algorithm ranking the prediction power through a backward selection. Starting with the most important variable to subdivide the sample, the other variables were ranked according to the importance (prediction power) criteria (Figure 6). Figure 6 clearly shows that dietary variables play an important role, nowithstanding the adjustment for all confounders. The 5 most important food variables ranked by RSF were again used in the traditional Cox regression (Table 4) mutually adjusted in the same model. The selection procedure by RSF identified a different set of variables compared to the regression backward selection. Interestingly, the RSF set included fatty meat, which was again significantly inversely related to risk despite different adjustments, as before.

Table 4. Cox regression model of mortality for food groups, selected foods, and a posteriori and priori food patterns, adjusted for covariates *.

Variables	HR * with Olive oil as Adjustment (95% CI)
Food groups (sum of frequencies)	(per one frequency per day, not mutually adjusted)
Legumes and vegetables (Legumi e vegetali)	1.07 (0.85 to 1.36)
Fresh cheese (Ricotta di pecora e di vacca, fiordilatte, mozzarella, provola affumicata)	**1.29 (1.03 to 1.63)**
Red meat (Carne rossa: carne magra e grassa)	0.89 (0.66 to 1.19)
Processed meat (Carni processate: salumi, salsicce, pancetta, guanciale, cotechino, zampone, prosciutto magro e grasso o cotto)	0.85 (0.70 to 1.03)
Fish and seafood (pesce e frutti di mare)	0.78 (0.57 to 1.07)
Sweets (Torte, crostate, cioccolata, prodotti confezionati)	0.89 (0.58 to 1.37)
First 5 foods after backward selection	(per one frequency per day, mutually adjusted)
Fatty meat (Carne grassa)	0.64 (0.39 to 1.06)
Fatty ham, baked ham (Carne grassa e cotta)	**0.59 (0.35 to 0.99)**
Meat sauce (Sughi di carne, ragù)	1.76 (0.97 to 3.20)
Sheep ricotta, fiordilatte, mozzarella, smoked provola (Ricotta di pecora, fiordilatte, mozzarella, provola affumicata)	**1.41 (1.04 to 1.92)**
Eggs (Uova)	**0.62 (0.41 to 0.94)**
First 5 RSF foods with highest importance	(per one frequency per day, mutually adjusted)
Semolina type and other bread (Pane bianco)	0.94 (0.84 to 1.04)
Pasta, rice, polenta (Pasta, riso, polenta)	0.93 (0.73 to 1.20)
Desserts (Dolci, crostate, etc.)	0.96 (0.62 to 1.50)
Fatty meat (Carne grassa)	0.63 (0.38 to 1.04)
Poultry, rabbit (Pollame, coniglio)	0.99 (0.65 to 1.50)
Components of PCA	(per pca-score, not mutually adjusted)
Energy-Rich Foods Pattern	0.96 (0.92 to 1.01)
Farmhouse Diet Pattern	**1.05 (1.00 to 1.10)**
Sweets Pattern	1.01 (0.95 to 1.08)
Winter Pattern	0.97 (0.92 to 1.02)
Elderly Pattern	1.01 (0.96 to 1.07)
A priori indices	(per index point, not mutually adjusted, excluding olive oil as covariate)
DASH	1.03 (0.97 to 1.10)
MedDiet score	0.98 (0.97 to 1.00)
MIND	0.96 (0.92 to 1.00)
Italian MedDiet index	0.95 (0.90 to 1.00)

Statistical significance is represented in bold. * Model corrected for sex (male, female), age (yrs), BMI (unit), education (low, medium, high), smoking (yes, no), comorbidity (≥2 vs. <2), wine (≥1 L/day vs. <1 L/day), olive oil, (extensive use vs. non-extensive use).

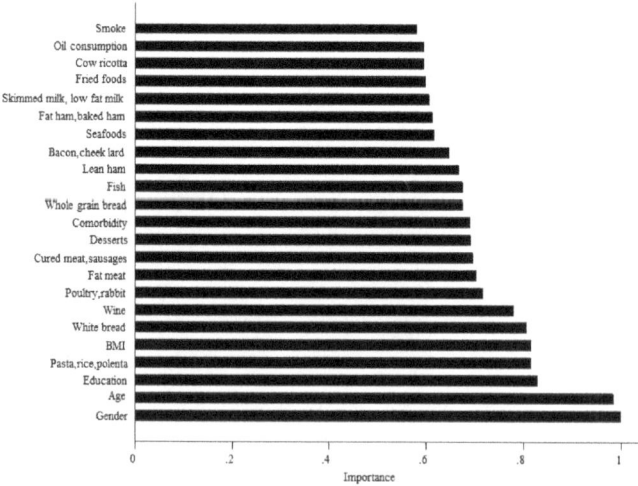

Figure 6. RSF, Importance score of predictor variables with covariates on all foods and olive oil with covariates on all foods and olive oil.

The relations of food patterns to risks of mortality are also shown in Table 4. Only the "Farmhouse Pattern" was significantly related to an increased risk of mortality. A decreased risk was associated with increasing scores for the Energy-Rich Food Pattern and the Winter Pattern, but this did not reach significance. The other two food patterns did not show any suggestive relationship to the risk of mortality.

Additionally, we investigated whether a priori healthy diet indexes such as the Meddiet score, Italian MedDiet Index, and the DASH and MIND indices were related to risk, created with the sum of the frequencies for each food included in the scores [8,17,22]. No significant association was found for the DASH index (HR 1.01, 95% CI 0.97 to 1.10). However, the MedDiet score, Italian MedDiet index, and the MIND index showed borderline inverse associations with risk of mortality (HR 0.98, 95% CI 0.97 to 1.00; HR 0.95 95% CI 0.90 to 1.00; HR 0.96, 95% CI 0.92 to 1.00, respectively).

In Table 5, we show the cause-specific results for the variables with significant associations with general mortality (Table 5). Not all of the variables showing associations with general mortality could be linked to the two causes of death, such as the "Farmhouse Diet" and fatty meat, fatty ham, and fresh cheese. However, we observed that eggs were inversely associated with risk of CVD death (HR 0.74, 95% CI 0.55 to 0.99) but not with cancer death (HR 0.85, 95% CI 0.65 to 1.10) (Table 5).

Table 5. Multiple Cox regression model of mortality, model adjusted *.

Parameters	Total Mortality	Cancer Mortality	Cardiovascular and Stroke Mortality
	HR (95% CI)	HR (95% CI)	HR (95% CI)
Components PCA §			
Farmhouse Diet Pattern	**1.05 (1.00 to 1.10)**	1.03 (0.93 to 1.13)	0.98 (0.88 to 1.10)
Foods §			
Fatty meat	0.89 (0.76 to 1.05)	0.97 (0.71 to 1.33)	0.79 (0.55 to 1.15)
Dairy products			
Sheep and cow ricotta, fiordilatte, mozzarella, smoked provola	**1.29 (1.03 to 1.63)**	1.42 (0.90 to 2.22)	0.96 (0.57 to 1.61)
Eggs	**0.86 (0.76 to 0.99)**	0.87 (0.66 to 1.13)	**0.73 (0.55 to 0.98)**
Fatty ham, baked ham	**0.59 (0.35 to 0.99)**	0.90 (0.35 to 2.32)	0.44 (0.14 to 1.45)

Statistical significance is represented in bold. Abbreviation: HR, Hazard Ratio; se(HR), standard error of HR; BMI, Body Mass Index; PCA, Principal Component Analysis. * Model corrected for: Sex (Female), Age (years), BMI, Education (Low, Medium, High), Smoking (yes), Comorbidity (≥ 2), Wine (≥ 1lt/day), and Olive oil, (No use or little) vs (Much use). § Parameters individually insert in the model.

4. Discussion

This prospective investigation carried out in a population-based cohort of 2472 Italian middle-aged participants of Castellana Grotte (Puglia Region, Italy) addressed dietary and other lifestyle factors and risk of mortality over a period of more than three decades. It appeared that traditional Mediterranean dietary variables such as fruit, vegetables, and fish were not associated with reduced individual mortality in this study population, but other dietary variables such as fatty meat and eggs were. The study also identified the "Farmhouse" pattern as positively associated with the risk of mortality. This pattern included, in particular, fresh cheese products that showed to be equally on the risky side of the analyses with food and food groups.

The study population of Castellana followed a traditional rural Mediterranean diet with a high frequency of consumption of fruit, vegetables alternating with legumes, a bread mostly based on a semolina type of meal, and local pasta. Whole bread was uncommon at the time of examination [11]. Most of the study population had attended school only for a few years and worked in the agricultural sector or in small enterprises. This might have led to a more uniform diet in terms of the major components. Other than this, traditional socioeconomic and lifestyle factors such as gender, low education, high BMI, and smoking showed an increased risk of mortality, even when mutually adjusted, confirming the internal validity of the study.

The Mediterranean lifestyle includes the consumption of wine, mostly at meals (nearly 11% of the population drank more than one liter per day), and olive oil as the traditional fat source (nearly 35% reported frequent use). Both types of lifestyle habits were taken into consideration in all dietary analyses as adjusting factors. Whereas heavy wine consumption did not increase the risk of mortality, probably due to lack of a detailed quantification of daily intake, the frequent use of olive oil showed a reduced association with risk compared to moderate and less use.

Olive oil has a remarkably strong effect on health, especially extra virgin olive oil (EVOO). EVOO is the dominant type of oil consumed in the rural area of Apulia, and is well-known to be related to a decreased risk of chronic diseases such as cardiovascular disease (CVD) and to cardiometabolic risk factors (inflammation, oxidative stress, coagulation, platelet aggregation, endothelial dysfunction, obesity, and type 2 diabetes mellitus) [23,24]. Dietary patterns, including olive oils, had been linked to a reduced risk of mortality in the Spanish and the Italian arms of the EPIC study [25]. The phenolic compounds of EVOO, such as hydroxytyrosol and oleuropein, are considered as the driving forces of the health implications of its use, and to a lesser extent, the composition of the fatty acids [26].

Despite the fact that none of the other food patterns was related to the risk of mortality, it is interesting to note that study participants with a diet more closely related to the "Energy-Rich Food" or the "Winter" patterns showed a tendency to a lower risk of mortality. These two patterns shared a high frequency of consumption of energy and protein-rich foods such as meat, white and red meat, chocolate, desserts, fish, seafood, legumes, and eggs, and had the semolina type of bread as a further source of energy in the form of carbohydrates. In this rural setting, the availability of dietary energy seemed to be a factor of individual survival. In line with these thoughts, the results of the food analyses identified fatty meats and eggs as associated with a lower risk of mortality. We do not claim a direct link of fatty meat with the risk of mortality but consider dietary energy as a potential indirect link. This type of food could also be linked with a fairly good economic situation. The finding regarding eggs appeared to be in accordance with the latest study results in the Mediterranean population. In view of the dietary cholesterol debate, it has been overlooked that eggs are a source of high-quality protein, vitamins of the B-complex, folate, fat-soluble vitamins, and several essential minerals. The EPIC study in Spain was the first that investigated egg consumption in a large free-living Mediterranean population. Despite their failure to find a relation with overall or specific cause mortality, they found an inverse relation with death due to nervous system alterations, predominantly Alzheimer's and Parkinson's diseases [27]. However, epidemiological data about the association between egg consumption and overall mortality is still limited, despite some reports of no link [28,29], particularly in Mediterranean populations.

Regarding specific causes of death, our results showed that a high frequency of consumption of eggs is associated with a reduced risk of death due to CVDs and stroke. In line with this finding, it is suggested that eggs may even promote some heart-healthy effects based on a study in which HDL cholesterol increased with the consumption of eggs during a moderate carbohydrate restriction in overweight individuals [30]. Otherwise, our finding regarding egg consumption is not corroborated in other studies and meta-analyses regarding stroke [29,31].

Milk and dairy products were part of the "Farmhouse" pattern and constitute an important source of energy as well as macro- and micronutrients in most Western countries; however, intakes differ largely between populations [32]. Study results regarding the long-term effects of those foods on health showed contradictory results [33,34]. This might be due to the fact that some studies were focused on the fat content of dairy products [35] and others on the impact of fermented and non-fermented dairy products [36,37]. Our results show that the consumption of non-fermented dairy products like sheep and cow ricotta, mozzarella, and smoked provola increased the risk of mortality, even after adjustment for other dietary factors. Similar results were reported by two other studies [38,39] conducted over the same time period in the Mediterranean area. Both investigations explored dietary habits in study populations in Greece. In this context, we should take the production process of such dairies, which requires salt, into account. In the late 1980s, the custom of making ricotta and cheese at home using milk local farming was still widespread in Puglia. A generous amount of salt was added to this dairy product [40]. Even in the current food composition tables prepared by the National Institute of Nutrition of Rome [41], 100 g of mozzarella contains around 200 mg of sodium (equal to 1.5 g of salt for a portion of 300 g) and smoked provola around 300 mg. We suppose that at the time of our data collection, it was common to use a much higher amount of salt in order to increase the palatability and shelf life of the products.

Advantages of this study include its long-term prospective observation (34-year follow up), the sample size, with a sufficient number of participants to address the research question, and the generalizability of the results to the south Italian population, the use of a larger number of foods to assess dietary habits, and the use of different statistical approaches.

The most important study limitation is the use of frequencies of foods instead of calculating quantitative daily intake. This type of measure could increase the bias that is usually associated with a retrospective dietary assessment over a period of a year, as compared to true intake, and also increase the bias that might be related to the risk estimates. To note, the survey questionnaire used in this study was not tested for its reliability and validity, and our results could have also been influenced by the subsequent changes in participants' dietary habits over the follow-up years since we used information from the first survey only. The assessment method could also be affected by lifestyle variables and socioeconomic status. In order to compensate for these influences, we always adjusted all dietary models for other lifestyle factors (sex, age, BMI, education, smoking, comorbidities, wine, and olive oil consumption). Sensitivity analyses were used in addition to considering confounding by other foods. Also, we limited the investigation to the most common causes of death. We cannot rule out the possibility of residual confounding by factors that have not been evaluated or are suboptimally measured. One of these factors could be the changing dietary habits, which partly occurred in this study population over time periods [11].

In conclusion, in this area of a prevalent Mediterranean diet, with high consumption of vegetables, legumes, and fruits, other dietary factors are driving individual survival. However, olive oil still appears to be a dominant food factor for decreased mortality. The traditional Mediterranean diet, together with high-energy foods, could explain the higher life expectancy of the Italian population according to our analysis. The issue of dairy foods remains controversial and is a topic warranting further investigation.

Author Contributions: Conceptualization, G.M.; Methodology: H.B., N.V., and V.G.; Software: F.C., V.G., and R.D.; Validation: V.G., R.D., and G.M.; Formal analysis: R.D. and V.G.; Investigation: G.M., L.L., I.B., and A.P.; Resources: R.S.; Data curation: V.G., R.D, and F.C.; Writing—Original Draft Preparation R.Z. and H.B.; Writing—Review and Editing, R.Z., H.B, R.S., F.P., and M.L.; Visualization, G.D.P., G.G., and H.B.; Supervision, G.D.P., G.G., and H.B.; Project Administration, G.G. All authors have read and agreed to the published version of the manuscript.

Funding: This research received no external funding.

Acknowledgments: We thank the MICOL Study group and the "Salus in Apulia" Research Team. This manuscript is the result of the research work on frailty undertaken by the "Italia Longeva: Research Network on Aging" team, supported by the resources of the Italian Ministry of Health—Research Networks of National Health Institutes. We thank the General Pratictionaires of Castellana Grotte, for the fundamental role in the recruitment of participants to this studies: Campanella Cecilia Olga Maria, Daddabbo Annamaria, Dell'aera Giosue', Giustiniano Rosalia Francesca, Guzzoni Iudice Massimo, Lomuscio Savino, Lucarelli Rocco, Mazzarisi Antonio, Palumbo Mariana, Persio Maria Teresa, Pesce Rosa Vincenza, Puzzovivo Gabriella, Romano Pasqua Maria, Sgobba Cinzia, Simeone Francesco, Tartaglia Paola, Tauro Nicola.

Conflicts of Interest: The authors declare no conflict of interest.

References

1. Wang, X.; Ouyang, Y.; Liu, J.; Zhu, M.; Zhao, G.; Bao, W.; Hu, F.B. Fruit and vegetable consumption and mortality from all causes, cardiovascular disease, and cancer: Systematic review and dose-response meta-analysis of prospective cohort studies. *BMJ* **2014**, *349*, g4490. [CrossRef] [PubMed]

2. Aune, D.; Keum, N.; Giovannucci, E.; Fadnes, L.T.; Boffetta, P.; Greenwood, D.C.; Tonstad, S.; Vatten, L.J.; Riboli, E.; Norat, T. Nut consumption and risk of cardiovascular disease, total cancer, all-cause and cause-specific mortality: A systematic review and dose-response meta-analysis of prospective studies. *BMC Med.* **2016**, *14*, 207. [CrossRef] [PubMed]
3. Mayhew, A.J.; De Souza, R.J.; Meyre, D.; Anand, S.S.; Mente, A. A systematic review and meta-analysis of nut consumption and incident risk of CVD and all-cause mortality. *Br. J. Nutr.* **2015**, *115*, 212–225. [CrossRef] [PubMed]
4. Zhao, L.-G.; Sun, J.-W.; Yang, Y.; Ma, X.; Wang, Y.-Y.; Xiang, Y.-B. Fish consumption and all-cause mortality: A meta-analysis of cohort studies. *Eur. J. Clin. Nutr.* **2015**, *70*, 155–161. [CrossRef]
5. Panagiotakos, D.B.; Pitsavos, C.; Stefanadis, C. Dietary patterns: A Mediterranean diet score and its relation to clinical and biological markers of cardiovascular disease risk. *Nutr. Metab. Cardiovasc. Dis.* **2006**, *16*, 559–568. [CrossRef]
6. Guenther, P.M.; Casavale, K.O.; Reedy, J.; Kirkpatrick, S.I.; Hiza, H.A.; Kuczynski, K.J.; Kahle, L.L.; Krebs-Smith, S.M. Update of the healthy eating index: HEI-2010. *J. Acad. Nutr. Diet.* **2013**, *113*, 569–580. [CrossRef]
7. Kant, A.K. Dietary patterns and health outcomes. *J. Am. Diet. Assoc.* **2004**, *104*, 615–635. [CrossRef]
8. Folsom, A.R.; Parker, E.; Harnack, L.J. Degree of concordance with DASH diet guidelines and incidence of hypertension and fatal cardiovascular disease. *Am. J. Hypertens.* **2007**, *20*, 225–232. [CrossRef]
9. D'Alessandro, A.; De Pergola, G. Mediterranean diet pyramid: A proposal for Italian people. *Nutrients* **2014**, *6*, 4302–4316. [CrossRef]
10. Zupo, R.; Lampignano, L.; Lattanzio, A.; Mariano, F.; Osella, A.R.; Bonfiglio, C.; Giannelli, G.; De Pergola, G. Association between adherence to the Mediterranean diet and circulating Vitamin D levels. *Int. J. Food Sci. Nutr.* **2020**. [CrossRef]
11. Veronese, N.; Notarnicola, M.; Cisternino, A.M.; Inguaggiato, R.; Guerra, V.; Reddavide, R.; Donghia, R.; Rotolo, O.; Zinzi, I.; Leandro, G.; et al. Trends in adherence to the Mediterranean diet in South Italy: A cross sectional study. *Nutr. Metab. Cardiovasc. Dis.* **2020**, *30*, 410–417. [CrossRef] [PubMed]
12. Attili, A.F.; Carulli, N.; Roda, E.; Barbara, B.; Capocaccia, L.; Menotti, A.; Okoliksanyi, L.; Ricci, G.; Capocaccia, R.; Festi, D.; et al. Epidemiology of gallstone disease in Italy: Prevalence data of the Multicenter Italian Study on Cholelithiasis (MI COL.). *Am. J. Epidemiol.* **1995**, *141*, 158–165. [CrossRef] [PubMed]
13. Misciagna, G.; Leoci, C.; Guerra, V.; Chiloiro, M.; Elba, S.; Petruzzi, J.; Mossa, A.; Noviello, M.R.; Coviello, A.; Minutolo, M.C.; et al. Epidemiology of cholelithiasis in southern Italy. Part II: Risk factors. *Eur. J. Gastroenterol. Hepatol.* **1996**, *8*, 585–593. [CrossRef] [PubMed]
14. Osella, A.R.; Misciagna, G.; Leone, A.; Di Leo, A.; Fiore, G. Epidemiology of hepatitis C Virus infection in an area of Southern Italy. *J. Hepatol.* **1997**, *27*, 30–35. [CrossRef]
15. World Health Organization. *Multimorbidity*; World Health Organization: Geneva, Switzerland, 2016; Available online: http://apps.who.int/iris/handle/10665/252275 (accessed on 19 July 2019).
16. Panagiotakos, D.B.; Pitsavos, C.; Arvaniti, F.; Stefanadis, C. Adherence to the Mediterranean food pattern predicts the prevalence of hypertension, hypercholesterolemia, diabetes and obesity, among healthy adults; the accuracy of the MedDietScore. *Prev. Med.* **2007**, *44*, 335–340. [CrossRef]
17. Morris, M.C.; Tangney, C.; Wang, Y.; Sacks, F.M.; Barnes, L.L.; Bennett, D.A.; Aggarwal, N.T. MIND diet slows cognitive decline with aging. *Alzheimer's Dement.* **2015**, *11*, 1015–1022. [CrossRef]
18. Agnoli, C.; Krogh, V.; Grioni, S.; Sieri, S.; Palli, D.; Masala, G.; Sacerdote, C.; Vineis, P.; Tumino, R.; Frasca, G.; et al. A priori-defined dietary patterns are associated with reduced risk of stroke in a large Italian cohort. *J. Nutr.* **2011**, *141*, 1552–1558. [CrossRef]
19. Smith, A.D.A.C.; Emmett, P.; Newby, P.K.; Northstone, K. Dietary patterns obtained through principal components analysis: The effect of input variable quantification. *Br. J. Nutr.* **2012**, *109*, 1881–1891. [CrossRef]
20. Ishwaran, H.; Kogalur, U.B.; Blackstone, E.H.; Lauer, M.S. Random survival forests. *Ann. Appl. Stat.* **2008**, *2*, 841–860. [CrossRef]
21. Dietrich, S.; Floegel, A.; Troll, M.; Kuhn, T.; Rathmann, W.; Peters, A.; Sookthai, D.; Von Bergen, M.; Kaaks, R.; Adamski, J.; et al. Random survival forest in practice: A method for modelling complex metabolomics data in time to event analysis. *Int. J. Epidemiol.* **2016**, *45*, 1406–1420. [CrossRef]
22. Panagiotakos, D.B.; Milias, G.A.; Pitsavos, C.; Stefanadis, C. MedDietScore: A computer program that evaluates the adherence to the Mediterranean dietary pattern and its relation to cardiovascular disease risk. *Comput. Methods Prog. Biomed.* **2006**, *83*, 73–77. [CrossRef] [PubMed]

23. Yubero-Serrano, E.M.; Lopez-Moreno, J.; Delgado, F.G.; Lopez-Miranda, J. Extra virgin olive oil: More than a healthy fat. *Eur. J. Clin. Nutr.* **2018**, *72*, 8–17. [CrossRef] [PubMed]
24. Guasch-Ferré, M.; Hu, F.B.; Martínez-González, M.A.; Fitó, M.; Bulló, M.; Estruch, R.; Ros, E.; Corella, D.; Recondo, J.; Gómez-Gracia, E.; et al. Olive oil intake and risk of cardiovascular disease and mortality in the PREDIMED Study. *BMC Med.* **2014**, *12*, 78. [CrossRef] [PubMed]
25. Masala, G.; Ceroti, M.; Pala, V.; Krogh, V.; Vineis, P.; Sacerdote, C.; Saieva, C.; Salvini, S.; Sieri, S.; Berrino, F.; et al. A dietary pattern rich in olive oil and raw vegetables is associated with lower mortality in Italian elderly subjects. *Br. J. Nutr.* **2007**, *98*, 406–415. [CrossRef] [PubMed]
26. Schwingshackl, L.; Lampousi, A.-M.; Portillo, M.P.; Romaguera, D.; Hoffmann, G.; Boeing, H. Olive oil in the prevention and management of type 2 diabetes mellitus: A systematic review and meta-analysis of cohort studies and intervention trials. *Nutr. Diabetes* **2017**, *7*, e262. [CrossRef]
27. Zamora-Ros, R.; Cayssials, V.; Clèries, R.; Redondo, M.L.; Huerta, J.; Rodríguez-Barranco, M.; Sánchez-Cruz, J.-J.; Mokoroa, O.; Gil, L.; Amiano, P.; et al. Moderate egg consumption and all-cause and specific-cause mortality in the Spanish European Prospective into Cancer and Nutrition (EPIC-Spain) study. *Eur. J. Nutr.* **2018**, *58*, 2003–2010. [CrossRef]
28. Guo, J.; Hobbs, D.A.; Cockcroft, J.R.; Elwood, P.C.; Pickering, J.E.; Lovegrove, J.; Givens, D.I. Association between egg consumption and cardiovascular disease events, diabetes and all-cause mortality. *Eur. J. Nutr.* **2017**, *57*, 2943–2952. [CrossRef]
29. Solfrizzi, V.; Agosti, P.; Lozupone, M.; Custodero, C.; Schilardi, A.; Valiani, V.; Santamato, A.; Sardone, R.; Dibello, V.; Di Lena, L.; et al. Nutritional interventions and cognitive-related outcomes in patients with late-life cognitive disorders: A systematic review. *Neurosci. Biobehav. Rev.* **2018**, *95*, 480–498. [CrossRef]
30. Mutungi, G.; Ratliff, J.; Puglisi, M.; Torres-Gonzalez, M.; Vaishnav, U.; Leite, J.O.; Quann, E.; Volek, J.S.; Fernandez, M.-L. Dietary cholesterol from eggs increases plasma HDL cholesterol in overweight men consuming a carbohydrate-restricted diet. *J. Nutr.* **2008**, *138*, 272–276. [CrossRef]
31. Rong, Y.; Chen, L.; Zhu, T.; Song, Y.; Yu, M.; Shan, Z.; Sands, A.; Hu, F.B.; Liu, L. Egg consumption and risk of coronary heart disease and stroke: Dose-response meta-analysis of prospective cohort studies. *BMJ* **2013**, *346*, e8539. [CrossRef]
32. Gerosa, S.; Skoet, J. Milk Availability: Trends in Production and Demand and Medium-Term Outlook. 2012. Available online: https://ageconsearch.umn.edu/record/289000/ (accessed on 12 December 2019).
33. Tognon, G.; Nilsson, L.M.; Shungin, D.; Lissner, L.; Jansson, J.-H.; Renström, F.; Wennberg, M.; Winkvist, A.; Johansson, I. Nonfermented milk and other dairy products: Associations with all-cause mortality. *Am. J. Clin. Nutr.* **2017**, *105*, 1502–1511. [CrossRef] [PubMed]
34. Deghan, M.; Mente, A.; Yusuf, S. Associations of fats and carbohydrates with cardiovascular disease and mortality-PURE and simple?—Authors' reply. *Lancet* **2018**, *391*, 1681–1682. [CrossRef]
35. Fontecha, J.; Juárez, M. Chapter 19—Recent advances in dairy ingredients and cardiovascular diseases with special reference to milk fat components. In *Dairy in Human Health and Disease across the Lifespan*; Watson, R.R., Collier, R.J., Preedy, V.R., Eds.; Academic Press: Cambridge, MA, USA, 2017; pp. 251–261. Available online: http://www.sciencedirect.com/science/article/pii/B9780128098684000194 (accessed on 12 December 2019).
36. Goulet, O. Potential role of the intestinal microbiota in programming health and disease: Figure 1. *Nutr. Rev.* **2015**, *73*, 32–40. [CrossRef] [PubMed]
37. Butel, M.-J. Probiotics, gut microbiota and health. *Med. Mal. Infect.* **2014**, *44*, 1–8. [CrossRef] [PubMed]
38. Trichopoulou, A.; Bamia, C.; Trichopoulos, D. Anatomy of health effects of Mediterranean diet: Greek EPIC prospective cohort study. *BMJ* **2009**, *338*, b2337. [CrossRef] [PubMed]
39. Trichopoulou, A.; Costacou, T.; Bamia, C.; Trichopoulos, D. Adherence to a Mediterranean diet and survival in a Greek population. *N. Engl. J. Med.* **2003**, *348*, 2599–2608. [CrossRef]
40. Guinee, T.P. Salting and the role of salt in cheese. *Int. J. Dairy Technol.* **2004**, *57*, 99–109. [CrossRef]
41. Carnovale, E.; Marletta, L. *Tabelle di Composizione Degli Alimenti*; Edra: Perignano, Italy, 1997; Available online: https://play.google.com/store/books/details?id=TfswAAAACAAJ (accessed on 12 December 2019).

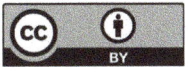

© 2020 by the authors. Licensee MDPI, Basel, Switzerland. This article is an open access article distributed under the terms and conditions of the Creative Commons Attribution (CC BY) license (http://creativecommons.org/licenses/by/4.0/).

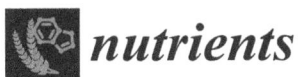

Review

Diet and Cardiovascular Disease Risk Among Individuals with Familial Hypercholesterolemia: Systematic Review and Meta-Analysis

Fotios Barkas [1,2], Tzortzis Nomikos [2], Evangelos Liberopoulos [1] and Demosthenes Panagiotakos [2,*]

1. Department of Internal Medicine, Faculty of Medicine, School of Health Sciences, University of Ioannina, 451 10 Ioannina, Greece; fotisbarkas@windowslive.com (F.B.); elibero@uoi.gr (E.L.)
2. Department of Nutrition & Dietetics, School of Health Science & Education, Harokopio University, 176 71 Athens, Greece; tnomikos@hua.gr
* Correspondence: dbpanag@hua.gr; Tel.: +30-210-9549332 or +30-210-9549100

Received: 17 July 2020; Accepted: 10 August 2020; Published: 13 August 2020

Abstract: Background: Although a cholesterol-lowering diet and the addition of plant sterols and stanols are suggested for the lipid management of children and adults with familial hypercholesterolemia, there is limited evidence evaluating such interventions in this population. Objectives: To investigate the impact of cholesterol-lowering diet and other dietary interventions on the incidence or mortality of cardiovascular disease and lipid profile of patients with familial hypercholesterolemia. Search methods: Relevant trials were identified by searching US National Library of Medicine National Institutes of Health Metabolism Trials Register and clinicaltrials.gov.gr using the following terms: diet, dietary, plant sterols, stanols, omega-3 fatty acids, fiber and familial hypercholesterolemia. Selection criteria: Randomized controlled trials evaluating the effect of cholesterol-lowering diet or other dietary interventions in children and adults with familial hypercholesterolemia were included. Data collection and analysis: Two authors independently assessed the eligibility of the included trials and their bias risk and extracted the data which was independently verified by other colleagues. Results: A total of 17 trials were finally included, with a total of 376 participants across 8 comparison groups. The included trials had either a low or unclear bias risk for most of the assessed risk parameters. Cardiovascular incidence or mortality were not evaluated in any of the included trials. Among the planned comparisons regarding patients' lipidemic profile, a significant difference was noticed for the following comparisons and outcomes: omega-3 fatty acids reduced triglycerides (mean difference (MD): −0.27 mmol/L, 95% confidence interval (CI): −0.47 to −0.07, $p < 0.01$) when compared with placebo. A non-significant trend towards a reduction in subjects' total cholesterol (MD: −0.34, 95% CI: −0.68 to 0, mmol/L, $p = 0.05$) and low-density lipoprotein cholesterol (MD: −0.31, 95% CI: −0.61 to 0, mmol/L, $p = 0.05$) was noticed. In comparison with cholesterol-lowering diet, the additional consumption of plant stanols decreased total cholesterol (MD: −0.62 mmol/L, 95% CI: −1.13 to −0.11, $p = 0.02$) and low-density lipoprotein cholesterol (MD: −0.58 mmol/L, 95% CI: −1.08 to −0.09, $p = 0.02$). The same was by plant sterols (MD: −0.46 mmol/L, 95% CI: −0.76 to −0.17, $p < 0.01$ for cholesterol and MD: −0.45 mmol/L, 95% CI: −0.74 to −0.16, $p < 0.01$ for low-density lipoprotein cholesterol). No heterogeneity was noticed among the studies included in these analyses. Conclusions: Available trials confirm that the addition of plant sterols or stanols has a cholesterol-lowering effect on such individuals. On the other hand, supplementation with omega-3 fatty acids effectively reduces triglycerides and might have a role in lowering the cholesterol of patients with familial hypercholesterolemia. Additional studies are needed to investigate the efficacy of cholesterol-lowering diet or the addition of soya protein and dietary fibers to a cholesterol-lowering diet in patients with familial hypercholesterolemia.

Keywords: diet; plant sterols; stanols; omega-3 fatty acids; familial hypercholesterolemia

1. Introduction

Familial hypercholesterolemia (FH) is the most common inherited metabolic disease caused by mutations of the genes involved in low-density lipoprotein cholesterol (LDL-C) catabolism and related with premature coronary heart disease (CHD) [1–3]. Considering the LDL-C reduction (over 50%) needed for the prevention against the development of cardiovascular disease (CVD) in such patients, lipid-lowering drugs are considered as their primary cardiovascular (CV) prevention therapy [4–6]. On the other hand, dietary interventions, such as the manipulation of fat content, increasing dietary intake of soluble fiber and increasing the intake of certain dietary components (i.e., soy protein, plant sterols and stanols, omega-3 fatty acids) are recommended in patients with FH who cannot start (i.e., children) or tolerate lipid-lowering therapy (i.e., statin intolerant patients) [6,7]. Nevertheless, the majority of these interventions have not been adequately investigated in such individuals and consensus has yet to be reached on the most appropriate dietary treatment for FH [8].

The aim of this work was to assess the CV efficacy of the currently recommended cholesterol-lowering diet and other forms of dietary intervention in children and adults diagnosed with FH.

2. Materials and Methods

2.1. Eligibility Criteria

2.1.1. Types of Studies

The present meta-analysis has been conducted according to the Preferred Reporting Items for Systematic Reviews and Meta-Analyses (PRISMA) (Table A1). Published randomized controlled trials (RCTs) were included in the present meta-analysis. Trials using quasi-randomization methods were alternatively included in case of sufficient evidence showing that treatment and comparison groups were comparable in terms of clinical and nutritional status.

2.1.2. Study Participants

Studies including children and adults with FH (alternative named as inherited dyslipidemia IIa) were considered eligible. Trials including patients with FH along with others not fulfilling the criteria of FH diagnosis were only included if the FH group was well defined and the results for these subjects were available.

2.1.3. Interventions

Cholesterol-lowering diet or any other dietary intervention aimed at serum total cholesterol (TC) or LDL-C reduction, for at least 3 weeks. RCTs comparing dietary treatment as a control with lipid-lowering drugs were excluded. However, we included those trials in which control and treatment groups differed only in diet. Trials comparing one form of modified dietary intake with another form of dietary intake were included in case of a head-to-head comparison.

2.2. Outcomes

Incidence and mortality of total CVD, CHD, stroke or peripheral arterial disease (PAD) were considered as the primary outcomes of interest in our meta-analysis. The secondary outcomes were the following: TC, triglycerides (TG), high-density lipoprotein cholesterol (HDL-C), LDL-C, very-low-density lipoprotein cholesterol (VLDL-C), apolipoprotein (apo) A-I, apoB and lipoprotein (a) (Lp(a)).

2.3. Information Sources

Relevant trials were identified by searching US National Library of Medicine National Institutes of Health Metabolism Trials Register (https://www.ncbi.nlm.nih.gov/pubmed) and clinicaltrials.gov.gr (https://clinicaltrials.gov) using the following terms: diet, dietary, plant sterols, stanols, omega-3 fatty acids, fiber and familial hypercholesterolemia. RCTs included in our analysis were also scrutinized for other trials fulfilling our eligibility criteria.

2.4. Data Collection and Analysis

2.4.1. Selection of Studies

At the initial stage of review and each update, two authors independently selected the trials which were eligible for inclusion in the present meta-analysis.

2.4.2. Data Extraction and Management

Two review authors (FB and DP) independently extracted data using an extraction form recording publication details, study population, randomization, allocation concealment, blinding, interventions and results of each trial. Any differences between them were resolved by consulting the other review authors (TN and EL).

Due to the different dietary interventions recommended in patients with FH, the included RCTs were divided into the following comparisons:

- Dietary interventions to reduce fat content.
- Supplementation with omega-3 fatty acids compared with placebo.
- Dietary interventions modifying unsaturated fat content.
- Cholesterol-lowering diet compared with dietary interventions increasing intake of plant stanols.
- Cholesterol-lowering diet compared with dietary interventions increasing intake of plant sterols.
- Dietary interventions increasing intake of plant stanols compared with plant sterols.
- Dietary interventions modifying protein content.
- Dietary interventions increasing intake of dietary fiber.

Outcome data were grouped into those measured at up to one, three, six, twelve months and annually thereafter. In case of outcomes recorded at other time periods (i.e., 2, 4, 6, 8 weeks), the authors examined them as well. Generally, a 4-week period is adequate to investigate the effects of dietary interventions on lipids. In order to assess how these effects were maintained, analyses at longer periods were preferred. For the primary outcomes, analyzing the results of longer follow-up would have been necessary.

In case of duplicate trials, we included the trial with the longest follow-up.

2.5. Assessment of Risk of Bias in Included Studies

We assessed the bias risk (low, unclear or high) of the following parameters: (i) sequence generation, (ii) allocation concealment, (iii) blinding (of participants, personnel and outcome assessors), (iv) incomplete outcome data addressed, (v) free of selective outcome reporting and (vi) free of other bias. Overall, trials were considered as high-risk if the majority of the evaluated parameters were considered at high or unclear bias risk. Any differences between FB and DP were resolved by consultation.

2.6. Measurements of Treatment Effect

No data were available regarding the incidence and mortality of CVD. In case of available data for these outcomes, the odds ratio (OR) and the corresponding 95% confidence intervals (CIs) would have been estimated.

Continuous outcomes were analyzed using the mean difference (MD) and associated 95% CIs. In case of different measurement scales, the standardized mean difference (SMD) was calculated. When only the standard error (SE) was available, it was converted to SD by being multiplied with the square root of the participant number.

2.7. Synthesis of Results

2.7.1. Missing Data

In order to allow an intention-to-treat analysis, the authors would have sought data on the number of participants with each outcome event, by allocated treatment group, irrespective of compliance and whether or not the participant was later thought to be ineligible or otherwise excluded from treatment or follow up.

RCTs not reporting the results of the FH subgroup have not been included in the present work. Although the authors were requested to supply this lacking data, no response was received at the time of writing this review.

2.7.2. Assessment of Heterogeneity

Heterogeneity between trial results was tested using a standard chi-square test ($p < 0.1$ was considered statistically significant) and I^2 statistic was used as a measure of heterogeneity [9]. The following ranges and descriptions were used: (i) 0–40%: might not be important, (ii) 30–60%: may represent moderate heterogeneity, (iii) 50–90%: may represent substantial heterogeneity and (iv) 75–100%: considerable heterogeneity.

2.8. Assessment of Reporting Biases

Publication bias was assessed with a funnel plot. Due to the lack of data on the primary outcomes, any secondary outcome reported by three or more trials was used for the funnel plot construction. Outcome reporting bias was assessed by comparing the original protocols of the included trials with the final published manuscripts. In case that the protocols were unavailable, the outcomes described in the Methods section of the final manuscripts were compared with the Results section to identify any outcomes not being reported. Finally, our clinical knowledge would help us identify any outcomes expected to be measured, but they were not reported.

2.9. Subgroup Analysis and Investigation of Heterogeneity

In case of observed statistically significant heterogeneity, a random-effect meta-analysis was performed. Otherwise, a fixed-effect model was used.

3. Results

3.1. Study Selection

As shown in Figure 1, of the 1430 references initially identified from the electronic and manual search studies, a total of 17 RCTs were included in the present meta-analysis.

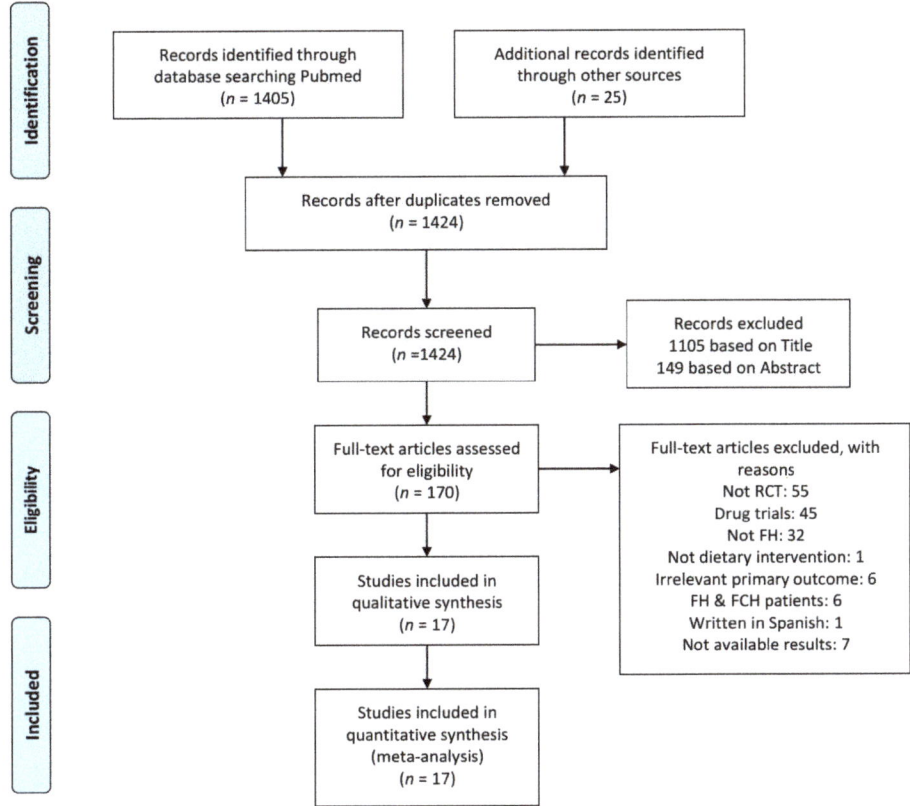

Figure 1. PRISMA flow diagram of study selection. FCH, familial combined hyperlipidemia; FH, familial hypercholesterolemia; RCT, randomized clinical trial.

3.2. Study Characteristics

The design of the RCTs included in the present meta-analysis, along with their samples and the investigated dietary interventions are demonstrated in Table 1. The majority of the included studies were double-blind, placebo-controlled and randomized with a cross-over design [7,10–15]. Their duration ranged from 3 to 13 weeks and their samples from 10 to 62 subjects. Seven trials enrolled children fulfilling the criteria of FH [10,12,14,16–19]. Among the rest studies including adults with FH, in 8 RCTs the subjects were also treated with lipid-lowering drugs [11,13,15,20–24].

Table 1. Characteristics of the included trials.

Trial	Study Design (Duration)	Participants	Interventions
Amundsen 2002 [10]	Double-blind, placebo-controlled randomized, cross-over (8w)	41 children with FH (aged 10.5 ± 1.7 yrs old, mean BMI 18.9 kg/m^2)	Low-fat/low-cholesterol diet and 1.60 ± 0.13 g plant sterols in a fortified spread (18.2 ± 1.5 g/d) vs. low-fat/low-cholesterol diet and placebo
Balestrieri 1996 [11]	Double-blind, randomized, cross-over (4w)	16 adults with FH treated with simvastatin (aged 45.2 ± 15 yrs old)	Cholesterol-lowering diet and 6 g/d fish oil ethyl ester vs. cholesterol-lowering diet and placebo (olive oil)

Table 1. Cont.

Trial	Study Design (Duration)	Participants	Interventions
Chan 2016 [20]	Open-label, placebo-controlled randomized, cross-over (8w)	22 adults with FH taking lipid-lowering therapy (aged 53.3 ± 3 yrs old, mean BMI 27 ± 1.4 kg/m^2)	4 g/d omega-3 fatty acid ethyl ester (46% eicosapentaenoic acid and 38% docosahexaenoic acid) vs. placebo
Chisholm 1994 [21]	Randomized, cross-over (8w)	19 adults with FH treated with simvastatin (aged 51 ± 10 yrs old, mean BMI 28.7 ± 1.2 kg/m^2)	Low-fat/low-cholesterol diet vs. a higher-fat/higher-cholesterol diet
De Jongh 2003 [12]	Double-blind, placebo-controlled randomized, cross-over (4w)	41 children with FH (aged 9.2 ± 1.6 yrs old, mean BMI 17.7 kg/m^2) and 20 controls (aged 8.2 ± 2.2 yrs old, mean BMI 17.5 kg/m^2)	Low-fat/low-cholesterol diet and 2.3 g plant sterols in a fortified spread (15 g/d) vs. low-fat/low-cholesterol diet and placebo
Fuentes 2008 [22]	Randomized, cross-over (4w)	30 adults with FH taking lipid-lowering therapy (aged 42 ± 18 yrs old, mean BMI 26.5 ± 3.7 kg/m^2)	4 low-fat diets with different content of cholesterol (<150 or 300 mg/d) and sitosterol (<1 or 2 g/d)
Gustafsson 1983 [25]	Randomized, cross-over (3w)	20 hyperlipoproteinemic adults: 6 with type IIa (aged 30–60 yrs old), 8 with type IIb (aged 41–65 yrs old) and 6 with type IV hyperlipoproteinemia (aged 51–66 yrs old)	2 low-cholesterol diets differing in polyunsaturated:saturated fat ratio (2.0 vs. 1.3)
Gylling 1995 [16]	Double-blind, placebo-controlled randomized, cross-over (6w)	14 children with heterozygous FH (aged 9.1 ± 1.1 yrs old, mean BMI 17.7 ± 0.9 kg/m^2)	Low-fat/low-cholesterol diet and 3 g sitostanol ester dissolved in rapeseed oil margarine vs. low-fat/low-cholesterol diet and placebo
Hande 2019 [13]	Double-blind, placebo-controlled randomized, cross-over (3m)	34 patients with FH on lipid-lowering treatment (aged 46.6 (18–71) yrs old, mean BMI 27.6 ± 5 kg/m^2)	4 g/d omega-3 fatty acids in a 1000 mg capsule consisting of 460 mg of eicosapentaenoic acid and 380 mg of docosahexaenoic acid (administered twice a day) vs. placebo (capsules with olive oil)
Helk 2019 [17]	Placebo-controlled randomized (13w)	26 children with FH (aged 8.7 ± 3.8 yrs old, mean BMI 16.3 ± 3.1 kg/m^2)	Diet high in unsaturated fats, low in saturated fats and enriched with soy-protein vs. diet high in unsaturated fats and low in saturated fats
Jakulj 2006 [14]	Double-blind, placebo-controlled randomized, cross-over (4w)	42 children with FH (aged 9.8 ± 1.5 yrs old, mean BMI 17.7 ± 2.8 kg/m^2)	Low-fat/low-cholesterol diet and 2 g plant stanols in a low-fat fortified yogurt (500 mL/d) vs. low-fat/low-cholesterol diet and placebo
Ketomaki 2005 [23]	Double-blind randomized, cross-over (4w)	18 adults with FH taking lipid-lowering therapy (aged 48 ± 2 yrs old)	Low-fat diet and 2 g plant stanols (25 g spread/d) vs. low-fat diet and 2 g plant sterols (25 g spread/d)
Laurin 1991 [18]	Randomized, cross-over (4w)	10 children with FH (aged 8 ± 1 yrs old, mean BMI 16.7 ± 0.9 kg/m^2)	2 different Low-fat/low-cholesterol/high-protein diets: about one-third (35%) of the protein energy was consumed as a dairy source, either from cow milk or a soy beverage
Negele 2015 [19]	Double-blind, randomized pilot trial (13w)	21 children with FH (aged 11.1 ± 3.4 yrs old, mean BMI: 19.1 ± 3.5 kg/m^2)	Low-fat/low-cholesterol diet and monounsaturated fatty acids by rapeseed oil vs. low-fat/low-cholesterol diet and polyunsaturated fatty acids by sunflower oil
Neil 2001 [15]	Double-blind, placebo-controlled randomized, cross-over (8w)	62 adults with heterozygous FH (30 were statin-treated) (aged 51.6 (33.3–62.3) yrs old, mean BMI 25.9 ± 3.5 kg/m^2)	Low-cholesterol diet and 2.5 g plant sterols in a fortified spread (25 g/d) vs. low-cholesterol diet and placebo
Wirth 1982 [24]	Randomized cross-over (2m)	12 adults with FH treated with fibrate (aged 51.7 (31–60) yrs old, mean BMI 26.6 kg/m^2)	Bezafibrate vs. bezafibrate and 5.2 g guar
Wolfe 1992 [26]	Randomized, cross-over (4-5w)	10 adults with familial hypercholesterolemia (2 of those had possibly FCH) (aged 50 ± 5 yrs old, with mean BMI 24.4 kg/m^2)	Low-fat/low-cholesterol/high-protein (23%) diet vs. low-fat/low-cholesterol/low-protein (11%) diet

BMI, body mass index; d, day; FCH, familial combined hyperlipidemia; FH, familial hypercholesterolemia; m, months; w, weeks; yrs, years.

We report on 8 dietary interventions separately.

- Only one study evaluated the impact of cholesterol-lowering diet in adults with FH, who were treated with simvastatin [21].
- Three trials compared the effect of treatment with omega-3 fatty acids in comparison with placebo [11,13,20]. The daily supplementation of omega-3 fatty acids was 5.1 g with a ratio of eicosapentaenoic acid/ docosahexaenoic acid (EPA/DHA) of 1:1 in the oldest trial [11], whereas the treatment arm in the rest RCTs comprised of 4 g/d of EPA/DHA (46% EPA and 38% DHA) [13,20]. All of these trials included adults taking lipid-lowering therapy [11,13,20] and only one reported that its subjects adhered to cholesterol-lowering diet [11].
- Two trials evaluated the impact of modified fat on FH patients. The former compared 2 low-fat diets enriched with either monounsaturated fatty acids (MUFAs) by rapeseed oil or polyunsaturated fatty acids (PUFAs) by sunflower oil in children with FH [19]. The second trial assigned its subjects to 2 cholesterol-lowering diets differing with regard to polyunsaturated:saturated values (2.0 and 1.3, respectively) [25].
- Two RCTs investigated the dietary interventions increasing the intake of plant stanols. The first study compared the addition of 3 g sitostanol dissolved in margarine to cholesterol-lowering diet with placebo in children with FH [16]. The second one evaluated the addition of 2 g plant stanols to cholesterol-lowering diet in a fortified yogurt in comparison with placebo in children with FH [14].
- Four trials evaluated the addition of plant sterols to cholesterol-lowering diet compared with placebo in FH patients [10,12,15,22]. Plants sterols were administered in a fortified margarine spread at a dose ranging 1.6-2.5 g/d. Two of the trials included children with FH [10,12] and the rest studies included FH adults receiving lipid-lowering drugs [15,22]. One trial compared the addition of 2 g/d plant stanols with 2 g/d plant sterols in FH adults who adhered to cholesterol-lowering diet and were on lipid-lowering therapy [23].
- Three RCTs evaluated dietary interventions modifying the protein content of the diet in FH patients [17,18,26]. Two of these trials manipulated protein content by increasing the consumption of soy protein [17,18]. The former compared 2 different cholesterol-lowering diets with high-protein content in which 35% of the protein was consumed as dairy source, either from soy beverage or cow milk [18]. The latter RCT investigated the addition of soy-protein to a diet high in unsaturated and low in saturated fats compared with placebo [17]. Both of these RCTs referred to children with FH [17,18]. The third trial investigated the increase in protein intake on top of a cholesterol-lowering diet in FH adults [26].
- Only one trial investigated the impact of dietary fibers on FH adults [24]. In this RCT, treatment with guar gum and bezafibrate was compared with bezafibrate alone [24]. The authors did not report whether their subjects adhered to cholesterol-lowering diet or not [24].

3.3. Bias Risk within Studies

The included trials had either a low or unclear bias risk for most of the parameters used for risk assessment (Figure 2).

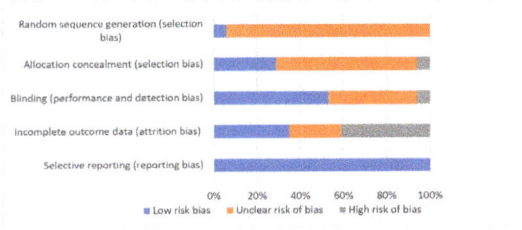

Figure 2. Bias risk graph. Judgments about each risk of bias item are presented as percentages across all included studies.

3.3.1. Allocation

Only one trial reported adequately on the randomization sequence; they stated that computer-generated random numbers were used for the assignment to either test or the control group with equal probability [15]. Reports on the generation of the randomization sequence were unclear in the remaining 16 trials [10–14,16–26].

Concealment of allocation was adequate in 5 trials where the methods used for allocation concealment were extensively described [12–15,19]. One trial was considered to be at high bias risk due its open-label design [20]. On the other hand, data regarding allocation concealment was unclear in the rest RCTs [10,11,16–18,21–26].

3.3.2. Blinding

Nine RCTs were reported as being double-blinded [10–16,19,23]. One RCT was open-label [20], whereas the rest trials did not provide any information regarding blinding [17,18,21,22,24–26].

3.3.3. Incomplete Outcome Data

It was unclear whether an intention-to-treat analysis was carried out in one of the trials, giving thus an unclear risk of bias [21]. Intention-to-treat analysis was adequate in 6 RCTs giving a low risk of bias [7,12,14,15,23,26]. In 7 RCTs participants were withdrawn and not included in the final analysis; consequently intention-to-treat analysis was not applied [10,11,13,18–20,22]. One trial undertook a per protocol analysis [17] and no sample attrition was performed in two RCTs [24,25].

3.3.4. Selective Reporting

No selective reporting was noted in the included RCTs.

3.4. Effects of Interventions

Only 11 RCTs presented data in such way that the preferred method of analysis could be conducted [10–18,20,22]. However, these trials did not provide data for all of the assessed outcomes. Furthermore, no RCT reported on the incidence or mortality of total CVD, CHD, stroke and PAD.

3.4.1. Dietary Interventions Reducing Fat Intake

Low-fat diet had no impact on subjects' TC (MD: −0.40 mmol/L, 95% CI: −0.95 to 0.15), TG (MD: 0.06 mmol/L, 95% CI: −0.43 to 0.55), HDL-C (MD: −0.11 mmol/L, 95% CI: −0.34 to 0.12), LDL-C (MD: −0.27 mmol/L, 95% CI: −0.79 to 0.25) and VLDL-C (MD: 0.01 mmol/L, 95% CI: −0.24 to 0.26), when compared with a higher-fat diet (Table S1) [21].

3.4.2. Supplementation with Omega-3 Fatty Acids Compared with Placebo

The lipid profile of subjects participating in the RCTs evaluating the administration of omega-3 fatty acids are demonstrated in Table S2 [11,13,20].

According to the pooled analysis (Figure 3), the supplementation with omega-3 fatty acids decreased study participants' TG (MD: −0.27 mmol/L, 95% CI: −0.47 to −0.07, p <0.01), but had no impact on their HDL-C (MD: −0.02 mmol/L, 95% CI: −0.16 to 0.12) and apoB100 (MD: −0.06 g/L, 95% CI: −0.18 to 0.06). A non-significant trend towards a reduction in subjects' TC (MD: −0.34 mmol/L, 95% CI: −0.68 to 0, p = 0.05) and LDL-C (MD: −0.31 mmol/L, 95% CI: −0.61 to 0, p = 0.05) was noticed (Figure 1). No significant heterogeneity was noticed across studies (Figure 3).

Total cholesterol

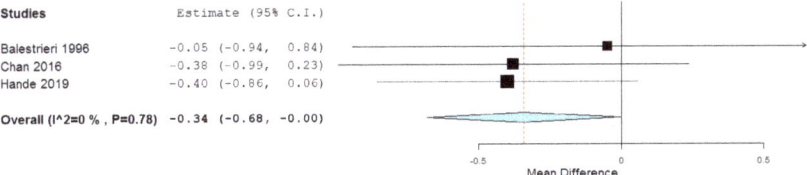

Triglycerides

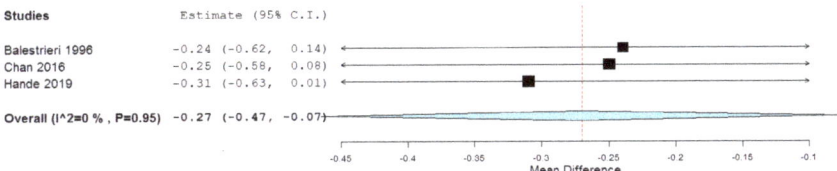

High-density lipoprotein cholesterol

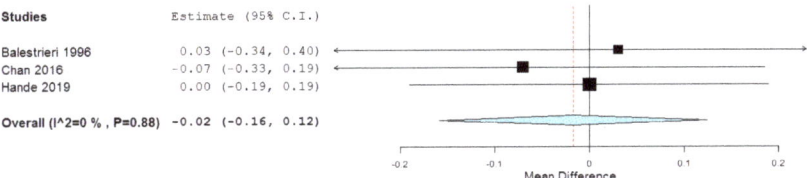

Low-density lipoprotein cholesterol

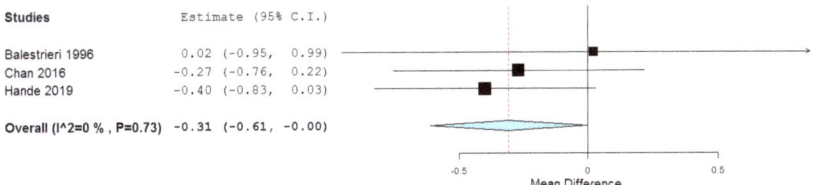

Apolipoprotein B100

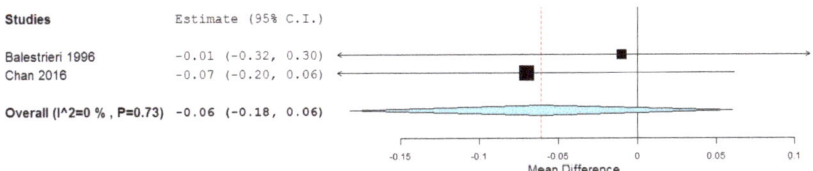

Figure 3. Effect of supplementation with omega-3 fatty acids compared with placebo.

Individual studies showed that omega-3 fatty acids decreased subjects' VLDL-C (MD: −0.20 mmol/L, 95% CI: −0.23 to −0.16, $p < 0.05$) [20], but no effect was noticed regarding their apoA-I (MD: 0.02 g/L, 95% CI: −0.31 to 0.35) and Lp(a) (MD: −0.02 g/L, 95% CI: −0.31 to 0.27) (Table S2) [11].

3.4.3. Dietary Interventions Modifying Unsaturated Fat Content

Low-Fat Diet Regimes Enriched with either Monounsaturated Fatty Acids or Polyunsaturated Fatty Acids

The trial comparing two low-fat diet regimes enriched with either MUFAs or PUFAs showed no difference between 2 groups regarding subjects' TC (MD: −0.73 mmol/L, 95% CI: −1.69 to 0.23), TG (MD: −0.03 mmol/L, 95% CI: −0.53 to 0.47), HDL-C (MD: 0.10 mmol/L, 95% CI: −0.19 to 0.39), LDL-C (MD: −0.84 mmol/L, 95% CI: −1.90 to −0.22), apoA-I (MD: −0.01 g/L, 95% CI: −0.25 to 0.23) and apoB100 (MD: −0.09 g/L, 95% CI: −0.36 to 0.18) (Table S3) [19].

Cholesterol-Lowering Diets Differing with Regard to Polyunsaturated:Saturated Values

One study showed that that increasing the PUFAs:saturated fat value of lipid-lowering diets from 1.3 to 2.0 did not offer a great advantage with regard to reduction in subjects' TC (0.03 ± 0.64 mmol/L), TG (−0.01 ± 0.23 mmol/L), HDL-C (0 ± 0.13 mmol/L), LDL-C (0.02 ± 0.06 mmol/L) and VLDL-C (0.09 ± 0.13 mmol/L) [25].

3.4.4. Cholesterol-Lowering Diet Compared with Dietary Interventions Increasing Intake of Plant Stanols

The lipid profile of subjects participating in the RCTs evaluating the dietary interventions increasing the intake of plant stanols are demonstrated in Table S4 [14,16].

According to the pooled analysis (Figure 4), the increased intake of plant stanols reduced study participants' TC (MD: −0.62 mmol/L, 95% CI: −1.13 to −0.11, $p = 0.02$) and LDL-C (MD: −0.58 mmol/L, 95% CI: −1.08 to −0.09, $p = 0.02$), but they had no impact on their TG (MD: −0.02 mmol/L, 95% CI: −0.09 to 0.14) and HDL-C (MD: −0.01 mmol/L, 95% CI: −0.11 to 0.09). No significant heterogeneity was noticed across studies (Figure 4).

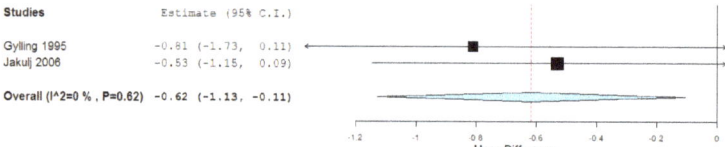

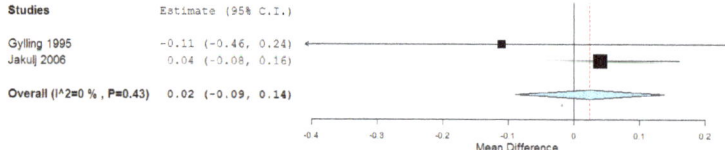

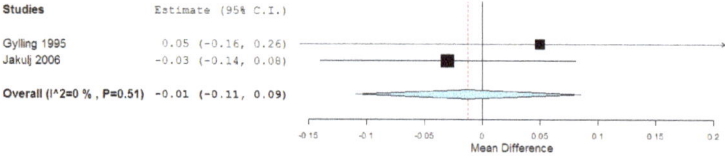

Figure 4. *Cont.*

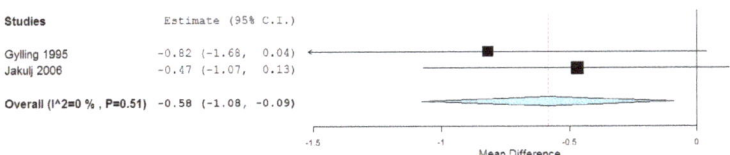

Figure 4. Effect of increased intake of plant stanols compared with placebo.

One study showed that plant stanols had no impact on subjects' VLDL-C (MD: −0.08 mmol/L, 95% CI: −0.26 to 0.10) (Table S4) [16].

3.4.5. Cholesterol-Lowering Diet Compared with Dietary Interventions Increasing Intake of Plant Sterols

The lipid profile of subjects participating in the RCTs evaluating the dietary interventions increasing the intake of plant sterols are demonstrated in Table S5 [10,12,15,22].

According to the pooled analysis (Figure 5), the increased intake of plant stanols reduced study participants' TC (MD: −0.46 mmol/L, 95% CI: −0.76 to −0.17, $p < 0.01$) and LDL-C (MD: −0.45 mmol/L, 95% CI: −0.74 to −0.16, $p < 0.01$). On the other hand, no effect was noticed regarding their TG (MD: −0.02 mmol/L, 95% CI: −0.13 to 0.09, HDL-C (MD: 0.02 mmol/L, 95% CI: −0.05 to 0.1,), apoA-I (MD: −0.03 g/L, 95% CI: −0.10 to 0.04) and apoB (MD: −0.06 g/L, 95% CI: −0.14 to 0.03) No significant heterogeneity was noticed across studies (Figure 5).

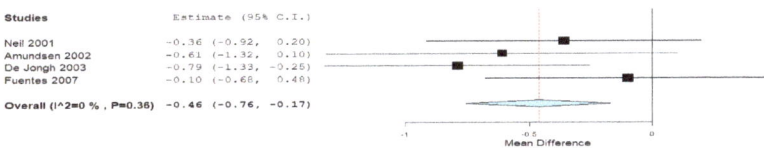

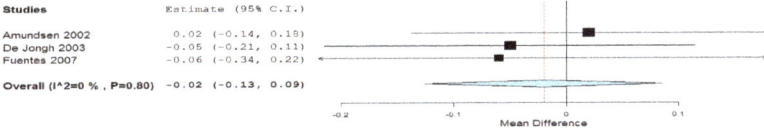

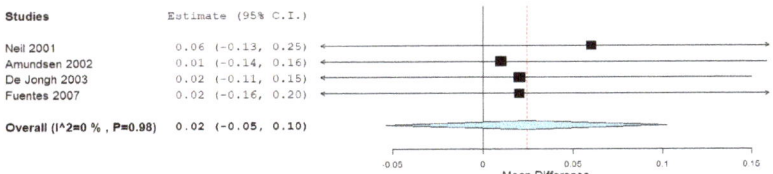

Figure 5. *Cont.*

Low-density lipoprotein cholesterol

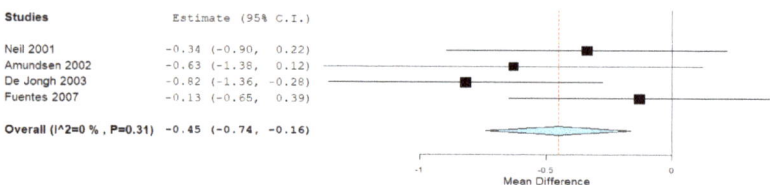

Apolipoprotein A-I

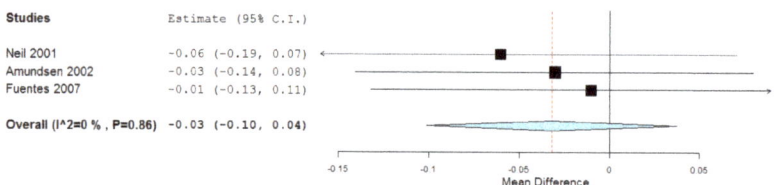

Apolipoprotein B

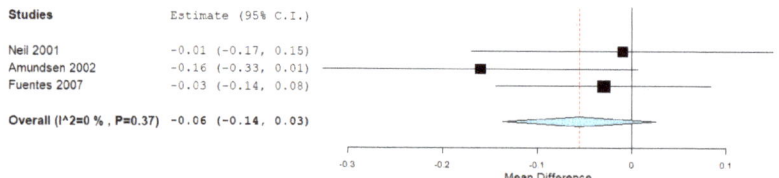

Figure 5. Effect of increased intake of plant sterols compared with placebo.

One study showed no impact on VLDL-C (MD: −0.08 mmol/L, 95% CI: −0.26 to 0.10) (Table S5) [15].

3.4.6. Dietary Interventions Increasing Intake of Plant Stanols Compared with Plant Sterols

There was no difference between the addition of 2 g/d plant stanols and 2 g/d plant sterols in FH adults who adhered to cholesterol-lowering diet regarding their TC (MD: −0.06 mmol/L, 95% CI: −0.66 to 0.54), TG (MD: 0.11 mmol/L, 95% CI: −0.18 to 0.40), HDL-C (MD: −0.05 mmol/L, 95% CI: −0.16 to 0.06) and LDL-C (MD: -0.05 mmol/L, 95% CI: −0.56 to 0.46) (Table S6) [23].

3.4.7. Dietary Interventions Modifying Protein Content

Soy Protein as a Form of Dietary Intervention Compared to Another Form or no Intervention

The lipid profile of subjects participating in the RCTs evaluating the dietary interventions increasing soy protein intake is demonstrated in Table S7 [17,18].

According to the pooled analysis (Figure 6), the dietary interventions increasing soy intake had no impact on study participants' TC (MD: −0.19 mmol/L, 95% CI: −0.78 to 0.41), TG (MD: −0.14 mmol/L, 95% CI: −0.30 to 0.02), HDL-C (MD: 0.08 mmol/L, 95% CI: −0.06 to 0.22L), LDL-C (MD: −0.41 mmol/L, 95% CI: −0.99 to 0.18), VLDL-C (MD: −0.06 mmol/L, 95% CI: −0.13 to 0.01), apoA-I (MD: −0.02 g/L, 95% CI: −0.10 to 0.05) and apoB (MD: −0.04 g/L, 95% CI: −0.14 to 0.06). No significant heterogeneity was noticed across studies, apart from the analysis concerning LDL-C (Figure 6).

Total cholesterol

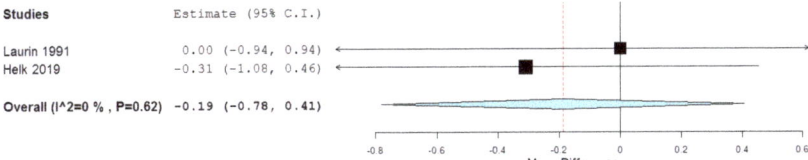

Triglycerides

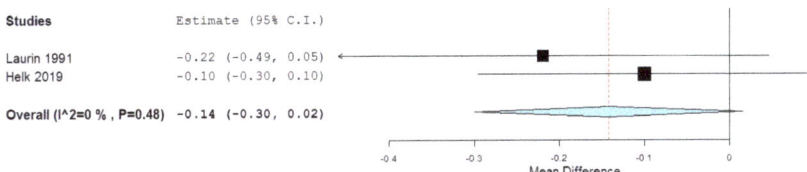

High-density lipoprotein cholesterol

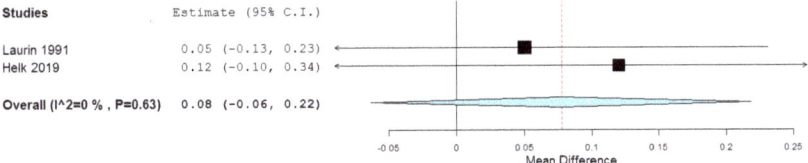

Low-density lipoprotein cholesterol

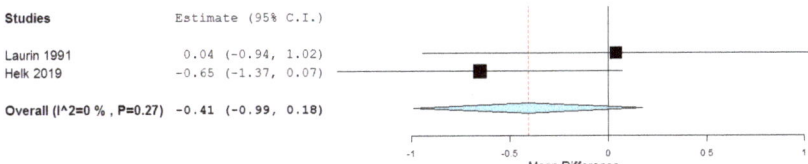

Very-low-density lipoprotein cholesterol

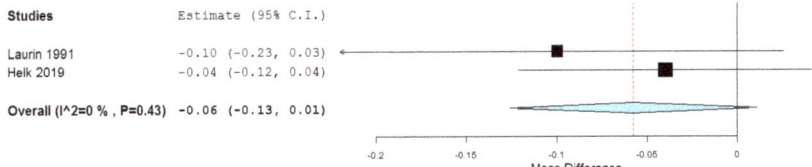

Figure 6. *Cont.*

Apolipoprotein A-I

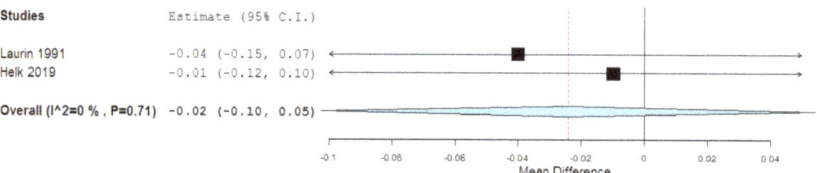

Apolipoprotein B

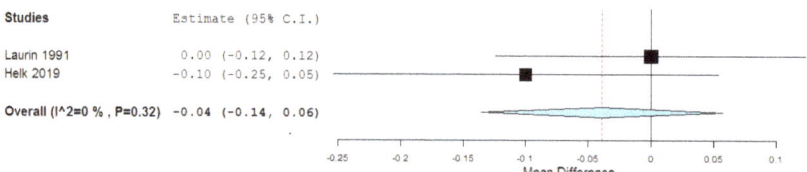

Figure 6. Effect of increased intake of soy protein compared with control group.

One study showed that soy had no impact on subjects' Lp(a) (MD: −0.29 g/L, 95% CI: −0.65 to 0.07) (Table S7) [17].

Dietary Intervention to Increase Protein Intake

The dietary interventions increasing protein intake reduced subjects' TG (MD: −0.70 mmol/L, 95% CI: −1.32 to −0.08, $p < 0.05$) and LDL-C (MD: −0.30 mmol/L, 95% CI: −0.85 to −0.25, $p < 0.05$), but had no impact on their TC (MD: −0.40 mmol/L, 95% CI: −1.23 to 0.43), VLDL-C (MD: −0.17 mmol/L, 95% CI: −0.44 to 0.10) and HDL-C (MD: 0.08 mmol/L, 95% CI: −0.14 to 0.10) (Table S8) [26].

3.4.8. Dietary Interventions to Increase Intake of Dietary Fiber

The dietary interventions increasing dietary fiber intake decreased subjects' LDL-C (MD: −1.83 mmol/L, 95% CI: −3.32 to −0.34, $p < 0.05$) and apoB (MD: −0.50 g/L, 95% CI: −0.65 to −0.35, $p < 0.05$). On the other hand, guar had no impact on their TC (MD: −0.57 mmol/L, 95% CI: −2.08 to 0.94), TG (MD: 0.41 mmol/L, 95% CI: −0.12 to 0.94), HDL-C (MD: −0.18 mmol/L, 95% CI: −0.47 to 0.11) and apoA-I (MD: 0.04 g/L, 95% CI: −0.05 to 0.13) (Table S9) [24].

4. Discussion

The present meta-analysis included 17 RCTs evaluating the impact of different dietary interventions on lipid levels of children and adults diagnosed with FH. No RCT investigating the impact of dietary interventions on CVD incidence or mortality was found. According to our pooled analyses, increased intake of plants sterols and stanols by fortified foods reduced TC and LDL-C in such individuals. Although a non-significant trend towards a reduction in TC and LDL-C was noticed, supplementation with omega-3 fatty acids resulted in TG decrease in this population.

FH is the most commonly inherited metabolic disease and associated with premature CVD, if left untreated [3–5,27,28]. Considering LDL-C reduction (over 50%) needed for the prevention against CVD development in FH patients, lipid-lowering drugs are the primary CV prevention therapy in such individuals [4–6]. Statins remain the cornerstone treatment and current guidelines recommend treating FH adults and FH children >8 years old with maximally tolerated doses of high-intensity statins, which are capable of lowering LDL-C ≥ 50% [4–6,29,30]. Ezetimibe and PCSK9 inhibitors are additional therapeutic options reducing LDL-C by 20–60%, in case that the patients are statin intolerant or do not achieve optimal LDL-C levels; of note, the latter has not been approved yet in children [4–6,29,30].

Novel lipid-lowering drugs, such as inclisiran, angiopoietin-like 3 protein, bempedoic acid and gemcabene are a few therapeutic options currently investigated for the future management of such individuals [5]. Despite the available effective lipid-lowering drugs, a considerable proportion of patients diagnosed with FH remain suboptimally treated in clinical practice [3,31]. In addition, there are patients diagnosed with FH who cannot be treated with lipid-lowering drugs, such as statin-intolerant or pregnant patients and children aged <8 years old [6]. In this context, dietary interventions including diet modification or dietary supplements might be helpful, if not necessary, in FH individuals. Indeed, current guidelines propose manipulating dietary fat, increasing fiber intake or certain dietary components for the management of patients with dyslipidemia, whereas phytosterols are recommended in hypercholesterolemic patients at low CV risk not qualifying for pharmacotherapy or as an adjunct to lipid-lowering therapy in those at high CV risk and in patients who cannot start (i.e., children or pregnant women with FH) or tolerate lipid-lowering therapy (i.e., statin intolerant patients) [6,7]. However, the majority of these interventions have not been adequately investigated in patients with FH.

Although cholesterol-lowering diet is the primary dietary suggestion in patients diagnosed with FH, only one study including FH adults has compared low-fat/low-cholesterol diet with a diet of higher content in fat and cholesterol and showed no difference between 2 interventions [21]. However, it has to be noticed that no data were available regarding the fat quality in subjects' diet [21]. Therefore, considering the fact that reduction of total fat intake is not so important as the modification of fat quality (i.e., replacement of dietary trans fatty acids with PUFAs) in CV prevention and cholesterol reduction [32,33], the results of Chisholm et al. are insufficient to reach any conclusion on the efficacy of cholesterol-lowering diet in FH patients. Increasing evidence has shown that FH individuals developing CHD exhibit risk factors associated with metabolic syndrome and insulin resistance, such as elevated TG, fasting blood glucose, obesity and hypertension or increased susceptibility to coagulopathy [34]. In this context, low-carb diet has been alternatively proposed over low-fat diet in FH patients with an insulin-resistant phenotype or increased thrombotic risk and the conduction of future trials assessing the effects of a low-carb diet on such individuals has been recently suggested [34]. As expected, the FH subjects of the included RCTs in the present analysis did not have increased TG or low HDL-C (Supplementary Materials), but the majority of the adult study participants were overweight (Table 1). Therefore, irrespectively of which diet will prove superior regarding the lipid management and CV prevention in FH patients, any dietary intervention reducing dietary intake is effective in weight reduction or control and should be recommended in such individuals, especially in those with overweight or obesity [35,36]. More importantly, diet should be a part of a holistic therapeutic plan ensuring patients' compliance and aiming at the improvement of CVD-related lifestyle factors, such as smoking, physical activity and body mass index control [37].

Similar to previous meta-analyses including dyslipidemic patients not fulfilling the criteria of FH [38], ours demonstrated that supplementation with omega-3 fatty acids significantly reduced TG, but had no impact on HDL-C levels of FH individuals. On the other hand, our results showing a non-significant trend towards a reduction in TC and LDL-C support the conflicting evidence regarding the impact of omega-3 fatty acids on cholesterol [38–40]. In this context, additional studies are needed to evaluate different quantity of EPA/DHA or quality of omega-3 fatty acids on FH patients' cholesterol indices. Indeed, REDUCE-IT trial which assigned its subjects to icosapent ethyl, a highly purified eicosapentaenoic acid ethyl ester or placebo showed that the former was associated with a significant non-HDL-C and apoB reduction [41]. Considering the fact that these are more accurate markers of the total atherogenic lipoproteins accounting for residual CVD risk than LDL-C [42], along with the fact that the insulin-resistant FH individuals are more prone to CVD development [34], omega-3 fatty acids could be beneficial in this subset of patients.

One trial comparing 2 cholesterol-lowering diets enriched with either MUFAs or PUFAs in FH patients did not confirm available evidence supporting that PUFAs may have a greater impact on LDL-C reduction than MUFAs [19,43]. Similarly, the replacement of saturated fat with PUFAs had no impact on FH patients' lipid profile in another study [25]. Nevertheless, the controversial results of these studies should be taken into account after considering the lack of data on their subjects' fat quality and the limitations regarding their small sample and design.

Undoubtedly, plant sterols and stanols are effective lipid-lowering dietary interventions and suggested by current guidelines for the management of dyslipidemias [44–46]. Not only our results confirmed previous evidence, but also showed that the cholesterol-lowering benefit of phytosterols seems greater in FH individuals; the average LDL-C reduction was 0.45–0.58 mmol/L in our analyses, whereas the corresponding reduction was 0.34 mmol/L in another one including RCTs with dyslipidemic individuals [44]. On the other hand, our results did not confirm available evidence supporting that phytosterols may also lower TG in normotriglyceridemic individuals [45,46].

Only one study has performed head-to-head comparisons between phytosterols in FH patients and showed no difference between 2 groups [23]. According to our results, a greater LDL-C reduction was noticed in the case of plant stanols rather than plant sterols (0.58 vs. 0.45 mmol/L). Despite not being significant, a similar trend was demonstrated by another meta-analysis including studies with hypercholesterolemic patients (MD: −0.13 mmol/L, 95% CI: −0.38 to 0.12, for the comparison between plant stanols and sterols) [44].

A regression analysis including a total of 312,175 participants from 49 RCTs with 39,645 major vascular events showed that bot statin and non-statin therapies (diet, bile acid sequestrants, ileal bypass and ezetimibe) were associated with similar risk ratios (RR) of major vascular events per 1-mmol LDL-C reduction (RR: 0.77, 95% CI: 0.71–0.84 for statins and RR: 0.75, 95% CI: 0.66–0.86 for non-statin therapies) [47]. Considering the linear association between LDL-C and CVD risk reduction noticed in that analysis, the addition of plant sterols or stanols lowering LDL-C by ~0.50 mmol/L in the FH patients would reduce their CVD risk by ~12.5% according to our results [47]. In addition, it has been proposed that phytosterols are cost-effective in reducing lifetime LDL-C burden in FH children [48]. Therefore, despite their small cholesterol-lowering effect, phytosterols could attenuate the efficacy of lipid-lowering drugs on CVD prevention in such individuals.

Our pooled analysis of 2 RCTs did not confirm the beneficial effect of increased soy consumption on cholesterol reduction [49]. However, it has to be noticed that apart from the limited number of the included RCTs in the analysis and their small sample, their control groups differed. The former compared 2 cholesterol-lowering/high-protein diets with increased intake of either soy protein or cow milk [18] and the latter compared a soy-enriched fat modified diet with a fat modified diet [17]. On the other hand, a small RCT demonstrated that increased protein intake decreased FH patients' LDL-C and TG [26]. Of note, no data were available regarding subjects' protein food sources. Therefore, future studies are needed in order to confirm the cholesterol-lowering effect of increased intake of soy protein in individuals diagnosed with FH.

Finally, the only RCT evaluating the impact of increased guar intake in FH patients has confirmed available evidence supporting the beneficial effect of dietary fiber on lipids [50,51].

Our results should be considered under certain limitations. First, only a few RCTs have investigated the impact of dietary interventions in patients with FH. Not only their samples were small, but also, they were short-term. In addition, the criteria for FH diagnosis was not defined in all studies and only almost half RCTs included patients taking lipid-lowering therapy. Finally, publication bias cannot be ruled out; there was no adequate data to assess selection, performance and detecting bias. However, a high-risk attrition bias was noticed. On the other hand, the present meta-analysis is the most recent to amplify the limited bibliography reporting on the impact of diet on FH patients [52–54]. Malhotra et al. were the last to perform a similar meta-analysis to ours in 2014 and confirm only the lipid-lowering effect of plant sterols on FH individuals [54]. In contrast to them, we included 7 additional RCTs in the present meta-analysis. Of note, a few methodological issues should be considered in the previous meta-analysis by Malhotra et al. Two RCTs included in their pooled analyses did not report separately on the subgroup of FH patients [55,56]. In addition, their pooled analysis evaluating the dietary interventions increasing the intake of plant stanols included 2 RCTs;

the former assigned their participants to plant stanols and placebo, but the latter assigned their subjects to plant stanols and plant sterols [16,57]. Finally, their pooled analysis evaluating protein intake included 2 trials with different dietary interventions. As already mentioned, Laurin et al. compared 2 low-fat/high-protein diets enriched by either soy protein or cow milk and Wolfe et al. compared a high- with a low-protein diet [18,26]. Therefore, our meta-analysis provides valuable data regarding the role of dietary interventions in CV prevention in FH patients. The addition of plant sterols and stanols to cholesterol-lowering diet, along with omega-3 fatty acids supplementation undoubtedly reduce cholesterol and TG in such individuals. However, future trials are needed to confirm the benefit of cholesterol-lowering diet and soy intake in this population. Last but not least, long RCTs are needed to elucidate the impact of such interventions on CVD incidence and mortality.

5. Conclusions

No robust conclusions can be reached about the impact of a cholesterol-lowering diet or any of the other dietary interventions proposed for FH patients on CVD incidence or mortality. Available RCTs confirm that the addition of plant sterols or stanols to low-fat diet has a cholesterol-lowering effect on such individuals. Considering their beneficial effect on lifetime LDL-C burden, phytosterols should be recommended in FH patients, especially in the children. On the other hand, supplementation with omega-3 fatty acids effectively reduces TG and might have a role in those exhibiting an insulin-resistant phenotype. Additional RCTs are needed to investigate the effectiveness of cholesterol-lowering diet and the addition of soy protein and dietary fibers to a cholesterol-lowering diet in patients with FH. Until then, physicians should keep in mind that diet aiming at weight reduction or control should be an integral part of a holistic approach aiming at the improvement of lifestyle CV risk factors.

Supplementary Materials: The following are available online at http://www.mdpi.com/2072-6643/12/8/2436/s1, Table S1. Lipid profile of subjects assigned to low-fat/low-cholesterol diet and high-fat/high-cholesterol diet. Table S2. Lipid profile of subjects assigned to omega-3 fatty acids and placebo. Table S3. Lipid profile of subjects assigned to low-fat diet regimes enriched with either monounsaturated fatty acids or polyunsaturated fatty acids. Table S4. Lipid profile of subjects assigned to plant stanols and placebo. Table S5. Lipid profile of subjects assigned to plant sterols and placebo. Table S6. Lipid profile of subjects assigned to plant stanols and plant sterols. Table S7. Lipid profile of subjects assigned to soy protein and control group. Table S8. Lipid profile of subjects assigned to increased and low protein intake. Table S9. Lipid profile of subjects assigned to bezafibrate plus guar and bezafibrate alone.

Author Contributions: Conceptualization, F.B. and D.P.; methodology, F.B.; software, F.B.; validation, T.N. and E.L.; formal analysis, F.B.; investigation, D.P.; resources, T.N.; data curation, E.L.; writing—original draft preparation, F.B.; writing—review and editing, T.N., E.L. and D.P.; visualization, T.N.; supervision, D.P. All authors have read and agreed to the published version of the manuscript.

Funding: This research received no external funding.

Conflicts of Interest: The authors declare no conflict of interest.

Appendix A

Table A1. PRISMA Checklist.

Section/Topic	#	Checklist Item	Reported on Page #
		TITLE	
Title	1	Identify the report as a systematic review, meta-analysis, or both.	1
ABSTRACT			
Structured summary	2	Provide a structured summary including, as applicable: background; objectives; data sources; study eligibility criteria, participants and interventions; study appraisal and synthesis methods; results; limitations; conclusions and implications of key findings; systematic review registration number.	1

Table A1. *Cont.*

Section/Topic	#	Checklist Item	Reported on Page #
		TITLE	
INTRODUCTION			
Rationale	3	Describe the rationale for the review in the context of what is already known.	2
Objectives	4	Provide an explicit statement of questions being addressed with reference to participants, interventions, comparisons, outcomes and study design (PICOS).	2
METHODS			
Protocol and registration	5	Indicate if a review protocol exists, if and where it can be accessed (e.g., Web address), and, if available, provide registration information including registration number.	N/A
Eligibility criteria	6	Specify study characteristics (e.g., PICOS, length of follow-up) and report characteristics (e.g., years considered, language, publication status) used as criteria for eligibility, giving rationale.	2
Information sources	7	Describe all information sources (e.g., databases with dates of coverage, contact with study authors to identify additional studies) in the search and date last searched.	3
Search	8	Present full electronic search strategy for at least one database, including any limits used, such that it could be repeated.	3
Study selection	9	State the process for selecting studies (i.e., screening, eligibility, included in systematic review, and, if applicable, included in the meta-analysis).	3
Data collection process	10	Describe method of data extraction from reports (e.g., piloted forms, independently, in duplicate) and any processes for obtaining and confirming data from investigators.	3
Data items	11	List and define all variables for which data were sought (e.g., PICOS, funding sources) and any assumptions and simplifications made.	3
Risk of bias in individual studies	12	Describe methods used for assessing risk of bias of individual studies (including specification of whether this was done at the study or outcome level), and how this information is to be used in any data synthesis.	3
Summary measures	13	State the principal summary measures (e.g., risk ratio, difference in means).	3–4
Synthesis of results	14	Describe the methods of handling data and combining results of studies, if done, including measures of consistency (e.g., I^2) for each meta-analysis.	4
Risk of bias across studies	15	Specify any assessment of risk of bias that may affect the cumulative evidence (e.g., publication bias, selective reporting within studies).	4
Additional analyses	16	Describe methods of additional analyses (e.g., sensitivity or subgroup analyses, meta-regression), if done, indicating which were pre-specified.	4
RESULTS			
Study selection	17	Give numbers of studies screened, assessed for eligibility and included in the review, with reasons for exclusions at each stage, ideally with a flow diagram.	4–5
Study characteristics	18	For each study, present characteristics for which data were extracted (e.g., study size, PICOS, follow-up period) and provide the citations.	5–7
Risk of bias within studies	19	Present data on risk of bias of each study and, if available, any outcome level assessment (see item 12).	8
Results of individual studies	20	For all outcomes considered (benefits or harms), present, for each study: (a) simple summary data for each intervention group (b) effect estimates and confidence intervals, ideally with a forest plot.	8–14
Synthesis of results	21	Present results of each meta-analysis done, including confidence intervals and measures of consistency.	8–14
Risk of bias across studies	22	Present results of any assessment of risk of bias across studies (see Item 15).	8–14
Additional analysis	23	Give results of additional analyses, if done (e.g., sensitivity or subgroup analyses, meta-regression (see Item 16)).	8–14

Table A1. *Cont.*

Section/Topic	#	Checklist Item	Reported on Page #
TITLE			
DISCUSSION			
Summary of evidence	24	Summarize the main findings including the strength of evidence for each main outcome; consider their relevance to key groups (e.g., healthcare providers, users and policy makers).	14–17
Limitations	25	Discuss limitations at study and outcome level (e.g., risk of bias), and at review-level (e.g., incomplete retrieval of identified research, reporting bias).	16–17
Conclusions	26	Provide a general interpretation of the results in the context of other evidence, and implications for future research.	17
FUNDING			
Funding	27	Describe sources of funding for the systematic review and other support (e.g., supply of data); role of funders for the systematic review.	17

N/A, Not applicable.

References

1. Austin, M.A.; Hutter, C.M.; Zimmern, R.L.; Humphries, S.E. Genetic causes of monogenic heterozygous familial hypercholesterolemia: A HuGE prevalence review. *Am. J. Epidemiol.* **2004**, *160*, 407–420. [CrossRef]
2. Vallejo-Vaz, A.J.; Kondapally Seshasai, S.R.; Cole, D.; Hovingh, G.K.; Kastelein, J.J.; Mata, P.; Raal, F.J.; Santos, R.D.; Soran, H.; Watts, G.F.; et al. Familial hypercholesterolaemia: A global call to arms. *Atherosclerosis* **2015**, *243*, 257–259. [CrossRef] [PubMed]
3. Barkas, F.; Liberopoulos, E.; Liamis, G.; Elisaf, M. Familial hypercholesterolemia is undertreated in clinical practice. *Hellenic J. Atheroscler.* **2016**, *7*, 120–130.
4. Goldberg, A.C.; Hopkins, P.N.; Toth, P.P.; Ballantyne, C.M.; Rader, D.J.; Robinson, J.G.; Daniels, S.R.; Gidding, S.S.; de Ferranti, S.D.; Ito, M.K.; et al. Familial hypercholesterolemia: Screening, diagnosis and management of pediatric and adult patients: Clinical guidance from the national lipid association expert panel on familial hypercholesterolemia. *J. Clin. Lipidol.* **2011**, *5*, S1–S8. [CrossRef]
5. Raal, F.J.; Hovingh, G.K.; Catapano, A.L. Familial hypercholesterolemia treatments: Guidelines and new therapies. *Atherosclerosis* **2018**, *277*, 483–492. [CrossRef] [PubMed]
6. Mach, F.; Baigent, C.; Catapano, A.L.; Koskinas, K.C.; Casula, M.; Badimon, L.; Chapman, M.J.; De Backer, G.G.; Delgado, V.; Ference, B.A.; et al. 2019 ESC/EAS Guidelines for the management of dyslipidaemias: Lipid modification to reduce cardiovascular risk. *Eur. Heart J.* **2020**, *41*, 111–188. [CrossRef]
7. Gylling, H.; Plat, J.; Turley, S.; Ginsberg, H.N.; Ellegard, L.; Jessup, W.; Jones, P.J.; Lutjohann, D.; Maerz, W.; Masana, L.; et al. Plant sterols and plant stanols in the management of dyslipidaemia and prevention of cardiovascular disease. *Atherosclerosis* **2014**, *232*, 346–360. [CrossRef]
8. Gidding, S.S. Special commentary: Is diet management helpful in familial hypercholesterolemia? *Curr. Opin. Clin. Nutr. Metab. Care* **2019**, *22*, 135–140. [CrossRef]
9. Higgins, J.P.; Thompson, S.G.; Deeks, J.J.; Altman, D.G. Measuring inconsistency in meta-analyses. *BMJ* **2003**, *327*, 557–560. [CrossRef]
10. Amundsen, A.L.; Ose, L.; Nenseter, M.S.; Ntanios, F.Y. Plant sterol ester-enriched spread lowers plasma total and LDL cholesterol in children with familial hypercholesterolemia. *Am. J. Clin. Nutr.* **2002**, *76*, 338–344. [CrossRef] [PubMed]
11. Balestrieri, G.P.; Maffi, V.; Sleiman, I.; Spandrio, S.; Di Stefano, O.; Salvi, A.; Scalvini, T. Fish oil supplementation in patients with heterozygous familial hypercholesterolemia. *Recenti Prog. Med.* **1996**, *87*, 102–105. [PubMed]
12. de Jongh, S.; Vissers, M.N.; Rol, P.; Bakker, H.D.; Kastelein, J.J.; Stroes, E.S. Plant sterols lower LDL cholesterol without improving endothelial function in prepubertal children with familial hypercholesterolaemia. *J. Inherit. Metab. Dis.* **2003**, *26*, 343–351. [CrossRef] [PubMed]

13. Hande, L.N.; Thunhaug, H.; Enebakk, T.; Ludviksen, J.; Pettersen, K.; Hovland, A.; Lappegard, K.T. Addition of marine omega-3 fatty acids to statins in familial hypercholesterolemia does not affect in vivo or in vitro endothelial function. *J. Clin. Lipidol.* **2019**, *13*, 762–770. [CrossRef] [PubMed]
14. Jakulj, L.; Vissers, M.N.; Rodenburg, J.; Wiegman, A.; Trip, M.D.; Kastelein, J.J. Plant stanols do not restore endothelial function in pre-pubertal children with familial hypercholesterolemia despite reduction of low-density lipoprotein cholesterol levels. *J. Pediatr.* **2006**, *148*, 495–500. [CrossRef]
15. Neil, H.A.; Meijer, G.W.; Roe, L.S. Randomised controlled trial of use by hypercholesterolaemic patients of a vegetable oil sterol-enriched fat spread. *Atherosclerosis* **2001**, *156*, 329–337. [CrossRef]
16. Gylling, H.; Siimes, M.A.; Miettinen, T.A. Sitostanol ester margarine in dietary treatment of children with familial hypercholesterolemia. *J. Lipid Res.* **1995**, *36*, 1807–1812.
17. Helk, O.; Widhalm, K. Effects of a low-fat dietary regimen enriched with soy in children affected with heterozygous familial hypercholesterolemia. *Clin. Nutr. ESPEN* **2020**, *36*, 150–156. [CrossRef]
18. Laurin, D.; Jacques, H.; Moorjani, S.; Steinke, F.H.; Gagne, C.; Brun, D.; Lupien, P.J. Effects of a soy-protein beverage on plasma lipoproteins in children with familial hypercholesterolemia. *Am. J. Clin. Nutr.* **1991**, *54*, 98–103. [CrossRef]
19. Negele, L.; Schneider, B.; Ristl, R.; Stulnig, T.M.; Willfort-Ehringer, A.; Helk, O.; Widhalm, K. Effect of a low-fat diet enriched either with rapeseed oil or sunflower oil on plasma lipoproteins in children and adolescents with familial hypercholesterolaemia. Results of a pilot study. *Eur. J. Clin. Nutr.* **2015**, *69*, 337–343. [CrossRef]
20. Chan, D.C.; Pang, J.; Barrett, P.H.; Sullivan, D.R.; Burnett, J.R.; van Bockxmeer, F.M.; Watts, G.F. Omega-3 fatty acid ethyl esters diminish postprandial lipemia in familial hypercholesterolemia. *J. Clin. Endocrinol. Metab.* **2016**, *101*, 3732–3739. [CrossRef]
21. Chisholm, A.; Sutherland, W.; Ball, M. The effect of dietary fat content on plasma noncholesterol sterol concentrations in patients with familial hypercholesterolemia treated with simvastatin. *Metabolism* **1994**, *43*, 310–314. [CrossRef]
22. Fuentes, F.; Lopez-Miranda, J.; Garcia, A.; Perez-Martinez, P.; Moreno, J.; Cofan, M.; Caballero, J.; Paniagua, J.A.; Ros, E.; Perez-Jimenez, F. Basal plasma concentrations of plant sterols can predict LDL-C response to sitosterol in patients with familial hypercholesterolemia. *Eur J. Clin. Nutr.* **2008**, *62*, 495–501. [CrossRef]
23. Ketomaki, A.; Gylling, H.; Miettinen, T.A. Non-cholesterol sterols in serum, lipoproteins, and red cells in statin-treated FH subjects off and on plant stanol and sterol ester spreads. *Clin. Chim. Acta* **2005**, *353*, 75–86. [CrossRef] [PubMed]
24. Wirth, A.; Middelhoff, G.; Braeuning, C.; Schlierf, G. Treatment of familial hypercholesterolemia with a combination of bezafibrate and guar. *Atherosclerosis* **1982**, *45*, 291–297. [CrossRef]
25. Gustafsson, I.B.; Boberg, J.; Karlstrom, B.; Lithell, H.; Vessby, B. Similar serum lipoprotein reductions by lipid-lowering diets with different polyunsaturated:saturated fat values. *Br. J. Nutr.* **1983**, *50*, 531–537. [CrossRef]
26. Wolfe, B.M.; Giovannetti, P.M. High protein diet complements resin therapy of familial hypercholesterolemia. *Clin. Invest. Med.* **1992**, *15*, 349–359.
27. Austin, M.A.; Hutter, C.M.; Zimmern, R.L.; Humphries, S.E. Familial hypercholesterolemia and coronary heart disease: A HuGE association review. *Am. J. Epidemiol.* **2004**, *160*, 421–429. [CrossRef]
28. Hutter, C.M.; Austin, M.A.; Humphries, S.E. Familial hypercholesterolemia, peripheral arterial disease, and stroke: A HuGE minireview. *Am. J. Epidemiol.* **2004**, *160*, 430–435. [CrossRef]
29. Barkas, F.; Liberopoulos, E.; Kei, A.; Makri, A.; Megapanou, E.; Pantazi, A.; Elisaf, M.; Liamis, G. Clinical application of PCSK9 inhibitors in a specialized lipid clinic. *HJM* **2018**, *120*, 229–237. [CrossRef]
30. Vuorio, A.; Kuoppala, J.; Kovanen, P.T.; Humphries, S.E.; Tonstad, S.; Wiegman, A.; Drogari, E.; Ramaswami, U. Statins for children with familial hypercholesterolemia. *Cochrane Database Syst. Rev.* **2017**, *7*, CD006401. [CrossRef]
31. Nordestgaard, B.G. Triglyceride-rich lipoproteins and atherosclerotic cardiovascular disease: New insights from epidemiology, genetics, and biology. *Circ. Res.* **2016**, *118*, 547–563. [CrossRef] [PubMed]
32. Judd, J.T.; Clevidence, B.A.; Muesing, R.A.; Wittes, J.; Sunkin, M.E.; Podczasy, J.J. Dietary trans fatty acids: Effects on plasma lipids and lipoproteins of healthy men and women. *Am. J. Clin. Nutr.* **1994**, *59*, 861–868. [CrossRef] [PubMed]

33. Lichtenstein, A.H.; Ausman, L.M.; Jalbert, S.M.; Schaefer, E.J. Effects of different forms of dietary hydrogenated fats on serum lipoprotein cholesterol levels. *N. Engl. J. Med.* **1999**, *340*, 1933–1940. [CrossRef] [PubMed]
34. Diamond, D.M.; Alabdulgader, A.A.; de Lorgeril, M.; Harcombe, Z.; Kendrick, M.; Malhotra, A.; O'Neill, B.; Ravnskov, U.; Sultan, S.; Volek, J.S. Dietary recommendations for familial hypercholesterolaemia: An evidence-free zone. *BMJ Evid. Based Med.* **2020**. [CrossRef] [PubMed]
35. Mansoor, N.; Vinknes, K.J.; Veierod, M.B.; Retterstol, K. Effects of low-carbohydrate diets v. low-fat diets on body weight and cardiovascular risk factors: A meta-analysis of randomised controlled trials. *Br. J. Nutr.* **2016**, *115*, 466–479. [CrossRef]
36. Gardner, C.D.; Trepanowski, J.F.; Del Gobbo, L.C.; Hauser, M.E.; Rigdon, J.; Ioannidis, J.P.A.; Desai, M.; King, A.C. Effect of low-fat vs. low-carbohydrate diet on 12-month weight loss in overweight adults and the association with genotype pattern or insulin secretion: The DIETFITS randomized clinical trial. *JAMA* **2018**, *319*, 667–679. [CrossRef]
37. Broekhuizen, K.; van Poppel, M.N.; Koppes, L.L.; Kindt, I.; Brug, J.; van Mechelen, W. Can multiple lifestyle behaviours be improved in people with familial hypercholesterolemia? Results of a parallel randomised controlled trial. *PLoS ONE* **2012**, *7*, e50032. [CrossRef]
38. Mozaffarian, D.; Wu, J.H. Omega-3 fatty acids and cardiovascular disease: Effects on risk factors, molecular pathways, and clinical events. *J. Am. Coll. Cardiol.* **2011**, *58*, 2047–2067. [CrossRef]
39. Ursoniu, S.; Sahebkar, A.; Serban, M.C.; Antal, D.; Mikhailidis, D.P.; Cicero, A.; Athyros, V.; Rizzo, M.; Rysz, J.; Banach, M.; et al. Lipid-modifying effects of krill oil in humans: Systematic review and meta-analysis of randomized controlled trials. *Nutr. Rev.* **2017**, *75*, 361–373. [CrossRef]
40. Pan, A.; Yu, D.; Demark-Wahnefried, W.; Franco, O.H.; Lin, X. Meta-analysis of the effects of flaxseed interventions on blood lipids. *Am. J. Clin. Nutr.* **2009**, *90*, 288–297. [CrossRef]
41. Bhatt, D.L.; Steg, P.G.; Miller, M.; Brinton, E.A.; Jacobson, T.A.; Ketchum, S.B.; Doyle, R.T., Jr.; Juliano, R.A.; Jiao, L.; Granowitz, C.; et al. Cardiovascular risk reduction with icosapent ethyl for hypertriglyceridemia. *N. Engl. J. Med.* **2019**, *380*, 11–22. [CrossRef] [PubMed]
42. Nordestgaard, B.G.; Langlois, M.R.; Langsted, A.; Chapman, M.J.; Aakre, K.M.; Baum, H.; Boren, J.; Bruckert, E.; Catapano, A.; Cobbaert, C.; et al. Quantifying atherogenic lipoproteins for lipid-lowering strategies: Consensus-based recommendations from EAS and EFLM. *Atherosclerosis* **2020**, *294*, 46–61. [CrossRef] [PubMed]
43. Astrup, A.; Dyerberg, J.; Elwood, P.; Hermansen, K.; Hu, F.B.; Jakobsen, M.U.; Kok, F.J.; Krauss, R.M.; Lecerf, J.M.; LeGrand, P.; et al. The role of reducing intakes of saturated fat in the prevention of cardiovascular disease: Where does the evidence stand in 2010? *Am. J. Clin. Nutr.* **2011**, *93*, 684–688. [CrossRef] [PubMed]
44. Demonty, I.; Ras, R.T.; van der Knaap, H.C.; Duchateau, G.S.; Meijer, L.; Zock, P.L.; Geleijnse, J.M.; Trautwein, E.A. Continuous dose-response relationship of the LDL-cholesterol-lowering effect of phytosterol intake. *J. Nutr.* **2009**, *139*, 271–284. [CrossRef]
45. Ras, R.T.; Geleijnse, J.M.; Trautwein, E.A. LDL-cholesterol-lowering effect of plant sterols and stanols across different dose ranges: A meta-analysis of randomised controlled studies. *Br. J. Nutr.* **2014**, *112*, 214–219. [CrossRef]
46. Rideout, T.C.; Chan, Y.M.; Harding, S.V.; Jones, P.J. Low and moderate-fat plant sterol fortified soymilk in modulation of plasma lipids and cholesterol kinetics in subjects with normal to high cholesterol concentrations: Report on two randomized crossover studies. *Lipids Health Dis.* **2009**, *8*, 45. [CrossRef]
47. Silverman, M.G.; Ference, B.A.; Im, K.; Wiviott, S.D.; Giugliano, R.P.; Grundy, S.M.; Braunwald, E.; Sabatine, M.S. Association between lowering LDL-C and cardiovascular risk reduction among different therapeutic interventions: A systematic review and meta-analysis. *JAMA* **2016**, *316*, 1289–1297. [CrossRef]
48. Vuorio, A.; Kovanen, P.T. Decreasing the Cholesterol Burden in Heterozygous Familial Hypercholesterolemia Children by Dietary Plant Stanol Esters. *Nutrients* **2018**, *10*. [CrossRef]
49. Jenkins, D.J.A.; Blanco Mejia, S.; Chiavaroli, L.; Viguiliouk, E.; Li, S.S.; Kendall, C.W.C.; Vuksan, V.; Sievenpiper, J.L. Cumulative meta-analysis of the soy effect over time. *J. Am. Heart Assoc.* **2019**, *8*, e012458. [CrossRef]
50. Jovanovski, E.; Yashpal, S.; Komishon, A.; Zurbau, A.; Blanco Mejia, S.; Ho, H.V.T.; Li, D.; Sievenpiper, J.; Duvnjak, L.; Vuksan, V. Effect of psyllium (Plantago ovata) fiber on LDL cholesterol and alternative lipid targets, non-HDL cholesterol and apolipoprotein B: A systematic review and meta-analysis of randomized controlled trials. *Am. J. Clin. Nutr.* **2018**, *108*, 922–932. [CrossRef]

51. Brown, L.; Rosner, B.; Willett, W.W.; Sacks, F.M. Cholesterol-lowering effects of dietary fiber: A meta-analysis. *Am. J. Clin. Nutr.* **1999**, *69*, 30–42. [CrossRef] [PubMed]
52. Poustie, V.J.; Rutherford, P. Dietary treatment for familial hypercholesterolaemia. *Cochrane Database Syst. Rev.* **2001**. [CrossRef]
53. Shafiq, N.; Singh, M.; Kaur, S.; Khosla, P.; Malhotra, S. Dietary treatment for familial hypercholesterolaemia. *Cochrane Database Syst. Rev.* **2010**. [CrossRef]
54. Malhotra, A.; Shafiq, N.; Arora, A.; Singh, M.; Kumar, R.; Malhotra, S. Dietary interventions (plant sterols, stanols, omega-3 fatty acids, soy protein and dietary fibers) for familial hypercholesterolaemia. *Cochrane Database Syst. Rev.* **2014**. [CrossRef]
55. Engler, M.M.; Engler, M.B.; Malloy, M.; Chiu, E.; Besio, D.; Paul, S.; Stuehlinger, M.; Morrow, J.; Ridker, P.; Rifai, N.; et al. Docosahexaenoic acid restores endothelial function in children with hyperlipidemia: Results from the EARLY study. *Int J. Clin. Pharmacol. Ther.* **2004**, *42*, 672–679. [CrossRef]
56. Nigon, F.; Serfaty-Lacrosniere, C.; Beucler, I.; Chauvois, D.; Neveu, C.; Giral, P.; Chapman, M.J.; Bruckert, E. Plant sterol-enriched margarine lowers plasma LDL in hyperlipidemic subjects with low cholesterol intake: Effect of fibrate treatment. *Clin. Chem. Lab. Med.* **2001**, *39*, 634–640. [CrossRef]
57. Ketomaki, A.; Gylling, H.; Miettinen, T.A. Removal of intravenous Intralipid in patients with familial hypercholesterolemia during inhibition of cholesterol absorption and synthesis. *Clin. Chim. Acta* **2004**, *344*, 83–93. [CrossRef]

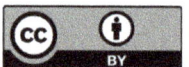

© 2020 by the authors. Licensee MDPI, Basel, Switzerland. This article is an open access article distributed under the terms and conditions of the Creative Commons Attribution (CC BY) license (http://creativecommons.org/licenses/by/4.0/).

MDPI
St. Alban-Anlage 66
4052 Basel
Switzerland
Tel. +41 61 683 77 34
Fax +41 61 302 89 18
www.mdpi.com

Nutrients Editorial Office
E-mail: nutrients@mdpi.com
www.mdpi.com/journal/nutrients

www.ingramcontent.com/pod-product-compliance
Lightning Source LLC
LaVergne TN
LVHW070556100526
838202LV00012B/482